Acute Pancreatitis

An A-Z

Acute Pancreatitis

An A-Z

V.K. Kapoor

Foreword
Hans G. Beger
Ulm, Germany

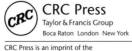

CRC Press
Taylor & Francis Group
Boca Raton London New York

CRC Press is an imprint of the
Taylor & Francis Group, an **informa** business

CRC Press
Taylor & Francis Group
6000 Broken Sound Parkway NW, Suite 300
Boca Raton, FL 33487-2742

© 2018 by Taylor & Francis Group, LLC
CRC Press is an imprint of Taylor & Francis Group, an Informa business

No claim to original U.S. Government works

Printed and bound in India by Replika Press Pvt. Ltd.

Printed on acid-free paper

International Standard Book Number-13: 978-1-138-89497-6 (Paperback)
978-1-138-09659-2 (Hardback)

This book contains information obtained from authentic and highly regarded sources. While all reasonable efforts have been made to publish reliable data and information, neither the author[s] nor the publisher can accept any legal responsibility or liability for any errors or omissions that may be made. The publishers wish to make clear that any views or opinions expressed in this book by individual editors, authors or contributors are personal to them and do not necessarily reflect the views/opinions of the publishers. The information or guidance contained in this book is intended for use by medical, scientific or health-care professionals and is provided strictly as a supplement to the medical or other professional's own judgement, their knowledge of the patient's medical history, relevant manufacturer's instructions and the appropriate best practice guidelines. Because of the rapid advances in medical science, any information or advice on dosages, procedures or diagnoses should be independently verified. The reader is strongly urged to consult the relevant national drug formulary and the drug companies' and device or material manufacturers' printed instructions, and their websites, before administering or utilizing any of the drugs, devices or materials mentioned in this book. This book does not indicate whether a particular treatment is appropriate or suitable for a particular individual. Ultimately it is the sole responsibility of the medical professional to make his or her own professional judgements, so as to advise and treat patients appropriately. The authors and publishers have also attempted to trace the copyright holders of all material reproduced in this publication and apologize to copyright holders if permission to publish in this form has not been obtained. If any copyright material has not been acknowledged please write and let us know so we may rectify in any future reprint.

Library of Congress Cataloging-in-Publication Data

Names: Kapoor, V. K. (Vinay Kumar), 1957- author.
Title: Acute pancreatitis : an A-Z / Prof. V.K. Kapoor.
Description: Boca Raton, FL : CRC Press, [2017] | Includes bibliographical references and index.
Identifiers: LCCN 2017000356| ISBN 9781138894976 (pbk. : alk. paper) | ISBN 9781315166759 (ebook)
Subjects: | MESH: Pancreatitis | Acute Disease | Handbooks
Classification: LCC RC858.P35 | NLM WI 39 | DDC 616.3/7--dc23
LC record available at https://lccn.loc.gov/2017000356

Visit the Taylor & Francis Web site at
http://www.taylorandfrancis.com

and the CRC Press Web site at
http://www.crcpress.com

Dedication

To
Professor Christian Herfarth

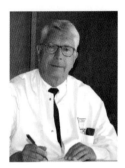

(*12 August 1933 in Breslau, †2 September 2014 in Heidelberg)

My professional host during my first visit abroad, when I visited the Chirurgische Klinik, University of Heidelberg, Germany, as a DAAD (German Academic Exchange Service) Fellow in 1991.

Contents

Foreword

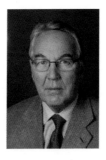

Diseases of the pancreas, particularly acute pancreatitis, are increasing in frequency worldwide. Additionally, two entities of diseases have been recently identified: autoimmune acute and chronic pancreatitis and cystic neoplastic lesions of the pancreas; both entities have links to acute pancreatitis. Since there is no specific medical treatment for acute pancreatitis, whether caused by biliary stone disease or by nutritional factors, e.g., alcoholic intoxication, knowledge about clinical understanding of acute pancreatitis and the respectively necessary and effective steps of management are extremely important. This book focuses on signal knowledge and on the best as well as fast clinical management of various facets of different types of acute pancreatitis.

Dr. Kapoor has produced a book about acute pancreatitis based on clinical evidence with the intention of a fast track program to manage mild as well as severe acute pancreatitis in the best manner possible.

Hans G. Beger
University of Ulm
Ulm, Germany

Preface

'Inflamed pancreas is a venomous snake which is best left untouched. Even a snake charmer should try to catch it only if he is sure to catch it.'

In the early 1980s, we opened up a patient with a clinical diagnosis of acute surgical abdomen and saw some mud (black, putty-like substance) in the upper abdomen—we did not know what it was and, obviously, what to do. The patient died.

In the mid-1980s, during an examination, I was asked to present a patient with a painful, tender, ill-defined upper abdominal mass in a sick-looking, septic patient. I had no clue as to what he had (I am sure neither did the examiners). I failed.

We know much more today about acute pancreatitis than we did in the 1980s and more patients are surviving and more examinees are passing.

Acute pancreatitis is a benign disease which is worse than cancer—for the patient to suffer from and for the doctor to manage.

Several text books of surgical gastroenterology and hepato-biliary-pancreatic surgery deal extensively with the topic, and many voluminous monographs have been written by the experts on the subject.

I have tried to put on paper what I understand about and how we manage our patients with acute pancreatitis, in a simple and easy-to-read format which anyone and everyone can understand.

The final word is, however, yet to be written about acute pancreatitis.

V.K. Kapoor
SGPGIMS
Lucknow, India

Acknowledgments

My views on the management of acute pancreatitis are based on the huge departmental experience with patients with acute pancreatitis referred to us. I am grateful to my faculty colleagues in the Department of Surgical Gastroenterology (Drs. S.P. Kaushik, Rajan Saxena, S.S. Sikora, Ashok Kumar, Anu Behari, R.K. Singh, Sujoy Pal, Anand Prakash, Biju Pottakkat, Ashok Kumar II, and Supriya Sharma); Department of Medical Gastroenterology (Late Dr. S.R. Naik and Drs. G. Choudhuri, V.A. Saraswat, Rakesh Aggarwal, U.C. Ghoshal, Praveer Rai, Samir Mohindra, Amit Goel, Abhai Verma, and Gaurav Pandey); Department of Radiology (Drs. S.S. Baijal, Archana Gupta, Sheo Kumar, Hira Lal, Zafar Neyaz, and Rajnikant Yadav); and the Department of Critical Care Medicine (Drs. A.K. Baronia, Banani Poddar, Afzal Azim, R.K. Singh, and Mohan Gurjar).

Thanks are due to Ms. Varsha Yadav and Mr. Pradeep Kumar for typing the manuscript.

Author

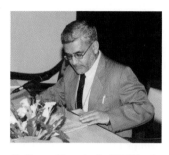

Dr. V.K. Kapoor is senior professor of surgical gastroenterology at the Sanjay Gandhi Postgraduate Institute of Medical Sciences (SGPGIMS), Lucknow, India. Prof. Kapoor has been a visiting professor at the Oregon Health and Science University (OHSU), Portland, OR, USA; the King's College Hospital (KCH), London, UK; and the International Medical University (IMU), Kuala Lumpur, Malaysia; and a visiting consultant surgeon at the Zayed Military Hospital (ZMH), Abu Dhabi, UAE. He is an examiner for the Intercollegiate MRCS at the Royal Colleges of Surgeons of England, Edinburgh, and Glasgow, UK, and has been an examiner at the University Kebangsan Malaysia (UKM), Kuala Lumpur, Malaysia; BP Koirala Institute of Health Sciences (BPKIHS), Dharan, Nepal; and the Health Authority of Abu Dhabi (HAAD), UAE. Dr. Kapoor has been awarded the Fulbright Fellowship, Commonwealth Fellowship, Scholarship of the International College of Surgeons, Clinical Oncology Fellowship of the UICC, and Fellowship of the German Academic Exchange Service (DAAD). He has also been awarded the Dr. B. C. Roy Award (Medical Council of India), International Fellowship (Indian Council of Medical Research), and Overseas Associateship (Department of Biotechnology). Prof. Kapoor has been an invited speaker at international conferences and at institutions in Australia, Austria, Bangladesh, Chile, China, the Czech Republic, the Dominican Republic, Egypt, France, Hong Kong, Hungary, Japan, Malaysia, Nepal, Oman, Pakistan, Poland, Singapore, South Korea, Sri Lanka, Thailand, Turkey, UAE, UK, and the USA.

ALSO BY THE AUTHOR

Kapoor VK. *Pearls in Surgery* (Foreword by Seymour I Schwartz). Hyderabad: Paras Medical Books; 2013:1–686. ISBN-13: 978-9383124022.

Kapoor VK, ed. *Surgery of Bile Ducts* (Foreword by Samiran Nundy). New Delhi: Elsevier; 2013: 1–172. ISBN 978-81-312-3397-9. Contributions from Japan, Netherlands, UK, and USA.

Kapoor VK. *Safe Cholecystectomy A-to-Z* (Foreword by John G Hunter). Lucknow: Shubham; 2010: 1–128. ISBN 978-81-910315-0-8.

Kapoor VK. *A–Z Pocketbook of Gall Bladder Cancer* (Foreword by LH Blumgart). New Delhi: Jaypee Brothers; 2010: 1–132. ISBN 978-81-8448-746-0.

Kapoor VK. *Venous Thrombo-Embolism (VTE) A-to-Z* (Foreword by V V Kakkar). Bangalore: Medeka Health; 2010: 1–99.

Abbreviations

AAA	abdominal aortic aneurysm
ABG	arterial blood gas
ACS	abdominal compartment syndrome
AGA	American Gastroenterology Association
AIP	autoimmune pancreatitis
ALT	alanine transaminase
AMI	acute mesenteric ischemia
ANA	antinuclear antibody
ANC	acute necrotic collection
APA	American Pancreatic Association
APACHE	acute physiological and chronic health evaluation
APFC	acute peripancreatic fluid collection
APS	American Pancreatic Society
ARDS	adult respiratory distress syndrome
ARF	acute renal failure
BMI	body mass index
BSI	blood stream infections
CAD	coronary artery disease
CAN	contrast-associated nephropathy
CBD	common bile duct
CCK	cholecystokinin
CCM	critical care medicine
CFTR	cystic fibrosis transmembrane
CHDF	continuous hemodiafiltration
CHF	congestive heart failure

CLD	chronic liver disease
CMV	cytomegalovirus
COPD	chronic obstructive pulmonary disease
CP	chronic pancreatitis
CRE	controlled radial expansion
CRI	catheter-related infections
CRP	C-reactive protein
CRRT	continuous renal replacement therapy
CT	computed tomography
CTSI	CT severity index
CVC	central venous catheter
CVP	central venous pressure
CVVHD	continuous venovenous hemodiafiltration
DIC	disseminated intravascular coagulation
DVT	deep venous thrombosis
EEUS	echo-enhanced US
EMD	erosive mucosal disease
EPC	European Pancreatic Club
EPF	external pancreatic fistula
EPT	endoscopic papillotomy
ERC	endoscopic retrograde cholangiography
ERP	endoscopic retrograde pancreaticography
ERCP	endoscopic retrograde cholangio-pancreatography
ETN	endoscopic transgastric necrosectomy
EUS	endoscopic ultrasonography
FFP	fresh frozen plasma
FJ	feeding jejunostomy
FNA	fine-needle aspiration
GI	gastrointestinal
GOO	gastric outlet obstruction
GS	gallstones
HAP	hospital-acquired pneumonia
HDU	high dependency unit
HES	hydroxyethyl starch
HU	hounsfield units
IAH	intraabdominal hypertension
IAP	International Association of Pancreatology
ICU	intensive care unit

IHBRD	intrahepatic biliary radical dilatation
IL	interleukin
IPMN	intraductal papillary mucinous neoplasm
IPN	infected pancreatic necrosis
IPPV	intermittent positive pressure ventilation
IVC	inferior vena cava
JVP	jugular venous pressure
LDH	lactate dehydrogenase
LFT	liver function tests
MAP	mean arterial pressure
MCN	mucinous cystic neoplasm
MD	multidetector
MDF	myocardial depressant factor
MI	myocardial infarction
MIPN	minimally invasive pancreatic necrosectomy
MIRN	minimally invasive retroperitoneal necrosectomy
MODS	multiple organ dysfunction syndrome
MOF	multiple organ failure
MRC	magnetic resonance cholangiography
MRCP	magnetic resonance cholangio-pancreaticogram
MRI	magnetic resonance imaging
MRP	magnetic resonance pancreaticography
NAC	N-acetyl-L-cysteine
NBM	nil by mouth
NOMI	nonocclusive mesenteric ischemia
NPI	nonpancreatic infections
PAF	platelet-activating factor
PAN	polyarteritis nodosa
PANCREA	Pancreatitis Across Nations Clinical Research and Education Alliance
PCA	patient-controlled analgesia
PCD	percutaneous catheter drain
PCEA	patient-controlled epidural analgesia
PCT	procalcitonin
PCWP	pulmonary capillary wedge pressure
PE	pulmonary embolism
PEEP	positive end-expiratory pressure
PMN	polymorphonuclear

PPC	pancreatic pseudocyst
PPI	proton pump inhibitors
PUD	peptic ulcer disease
RAP	recurrent acute pancreatitis
SCFA	short-chain fatty acids
SGD	selective gut decontamination
SIMV	synchronized (effort triggered) intermittent mandatory ventilation
SIRS	systemic inflammatory response syndrome
SLE	systemic lupus erythematosus
SPINK	serine protease inhibitor kajal
SSAT	Society for Surgery of the Alimentary Tract
SVE	side-viewing endoscopy
SVT	splenic vein thrombosis
TAP	trypsinogen-activation peptide
TDS	transduodenal sphincteroplasty
TNF	tumor necrosis factor
TPN	total parenteral nutrition
UGIE	upper gastrointestinal endoscope
US	ultrasonography
UTI	urinary tract infection
VAP	ventilator-associated pneumonia
VARD	video-assisted retroperitoneal debridement
VTE	venous thromboembolism
WON	walled-off necrosis

Key points about acute pancreatitis

- Sudden onset severe upper abdominal pain should raise a suspicion of acute pancreatitis.
- Surgical causes must be ruled out before a diagnosis of acute pancreatitis is made in a patient with upper acute abdomen.
- The majority of patients have mild acute pancreatitis that settles with conservative management in a few days' time.
- Patients with moderate or severe acute pancreatitis should be managed jointly by a team of physician/gastroenterologist/endoscopist, surgeon, and intensivist in HDU/ICU (with the backing of an interventional radiologist).
- Contrast-enhanced CT scan should be obtained around Day 5–7 of the attack of severe acute pancreatitis to detect necrosis.
- Infection of necrosis is the key factor for outcome.
- Use of prophylactic antibiotics in severe acute pancreatitis is controversial—most physicians, however, give them.
- Early and aggressive enteral nutrition is not only harmless but also beneficial.
- Percutaneous radiological intervention in the form of catheter drainage may buy time and delay surgery.
- Endoscopy plays an important role in the management of a pseudocyst.

- Surgical intervention should be delayed as long as possible; it should be minimally invasive rather than an open surgical procedure.
- The cause of acute pancreatitis should be established and preventive measures taken to avoid a repeat attack.

God put the pancreas in the back because he or she did not want surgeons messing with it.

A

A&E

Most patients with acute pancreatitis will present to the Accident and Emergency (A&E) Unit with sudden onset abdomen pain and will therefore be first seen by the emergency physician and the resident doctor on call. Those working in A&E should therefore be familiar with clinical presentation, diagnosis, and initial management of acute pancreatitis.

ABDOMINAL AORTIC ANEURYSM (AAA)

Patients with AAA can present as an acute abdomen, i.e., sudden onset severe persistent central upper abdomen (or lower chest) pain, which may sometimes be perceived by the patient as backache, because of one of its complications, viz., leak or rupture, and can mimic acute pancreatitis. Suspicion of an abdominal aortic catastrophe, viz., leaking or ruptured aneurysm or **aortic dissection**, is one of the indications for early, i.e., at the time of admission, contrast-enhanced CT in acute pancreatitis.

AAA is commonly seen in elderly smoker men. A pulsatile epigastric or periumbilical lump with bruit may be palpable; absence of a palpable pulsatile abdominal lump, however, does not rule out the diagnosis of AAA. The aneurysm can be picked up on Doppler ultrasonography (US), but contrast-enhanced CT or MR angiography is the diagnostic investigation.

Leak and rupture are two stages of the same disease process. A leaking AAA in a hemodynamically stable patient allows time for investigations and can be handled by endovascular aneurysm repair. A ruptured AAA with hemodynamic instability needs an immediate laparotomy and surgical repair of the aneurysm.

A # ABDOMINAL COMPARTMENT SYNDROME (ACS)

Patients with acute pancreatitis may develop intraabdominal hypertension (IAH) (intraabdominal pressure >12–15 mm Hg) and develop abdominal compartment syndrome (ACS) (intraabdominal pressure >20–25 mm Hg associated with new onset organ failure) due to edema of organs, mesentery, retroperitoneum and abdominal wall, and paralytic ileus.

Intraabdominal pressure is measured by a urinary bladder catheter using pubic symphysis as the reference 0 (zero).

ACS can cause multiple organ dysfunction such as

1. Decreased venous return caused by pressure on the inferior vena cava (IVC), resulting in decreased cardiac output
2. Restricted ventilation due to raised domes of the diaphragm, leading to **hypoxia** and hypercarbia
3. Impaired renal perfusion and renal dysfunction
4. Increased intracranial pressure (ICP)
5. Reduced mesenteric blood flow, causing **translocation** of bacteria across the bowel wall
6. Poor healing of abdominal wound

Management of ACS includes nasogastric decompression, rectal decompression with flatus tube or endoscope, fluid restriction, ultrafiltration/dieresis, adequate analgesia, and sedation to decrease abdominal muscle tone and prokinetics. Sustained intraabdominal pressure >20–25 mm Hg with new onset organ failure is an indication for intervention including percutaneous catheter drainage (PCD) of ascites, subcutaneous fasciotomy in anterior abdominal wall, and decompression laparotomy and laparostomy with mesh. In case of a difficult abdominal closure, laparostomy with a sterile urobag stitched to the wound edges (to prevent evisceration and dehydration of bowel loops) is an option. Surgical intervention is rarely required for ACS.

ACS is important—there is even a World Society of ACS! (https://www.wsacs.org/).

ABDOMINAL X-RAYS

Plain X-rays of the abdomen are not of much help in the diagnosis of acute pancreatitis but are more useful to rule out other causes of **acute abdomen**, e.g., intestinal obstruction and perforation peritonitis (Figure A.1). In patients with acute pancreatitis, plain X-rays of the abdomen may show a sentinel jejunal loop, dilated proximal transverse colon with cut off, and obscure psoas margins. Presence of pancreatic calcification suggests underlying **chronic pancreatitis** with superimposed attack of acute pancreatitis.

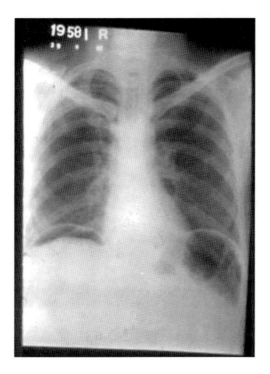

Figure A.1 X-ray chest showing free air under the right dome of diaphragm.

A

ABGs (ARTERIAL BLOOD GASES)

ABGs should be done in patients with acute pancreatitis to detect **hypoxia**, **hypercarbia**, and **acidosis** as early signs of impending respiratory failure as a component of multiple organ dysfunction syndrome (MODS).

ABSCESS, PANCREATIC

(Peri)pancreatic abscess is a well-localized, circumscribed collection of pus (but may also contain variable amounts of solid necrotic debris) with a mature wall (cf. acute peripancreatic fluid collection [APFC], which has no wall; cf. pseudocyst, which contains fluid). This may evolve from infection of an APFC or pseudocyst following acute pancreatitis (when contents are mainly pus and easily amenable to PCD) or from liquefaction of peripancreatic **necrosis** (when contents are both pus and solid necrotic debris and may require surgical evacuation).

Abscess usually forms 4 weeks after the onset of acute pancreatitis. Patients with pancreatic abscess have fever, **leucocytosis**, and a tender lump (cf. pseudocyst—no fever, no leucocytosis, and non-tender lump). US and CT show a thick-walled lesion with heterogeneous contents (Figure A.2), i.e., pus and debris (Figure A.3).

An abscess may erode into the adjacent bowel (spontaneous resolution) or vessel (resulting in **pseudoaneurysm**).

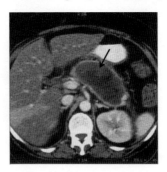

Figure A.2 CT showing pancreatic **abscess**—well localized, thick walled, and containing thick material.

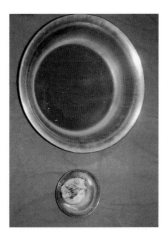

Figure A.3 More pus and little necrotic debris in pancreatic **abscess**.

Pancreatic abscess can be drained percutaneously (with US or CT guidance) or surgically (laparoscopic or open operation). PCD is the treatment of choice; surgical drainage may be required for multiple or multiseptate abscesses or for those not responding to PCD.

The revised Atlanta classification has omitted the term "abscess." APFC, acute necrotic collection (ANC), pancreatic pseudocyst (PPC), and walled-off necrosis (WON) may all get infected. The author is of the opinion that the term pancreatic abscess should be retained to include patients with a loculated collection of infected fluid or necrosis with systemic sepsis.

See also **Intraabdominal abscess**.

ACCESS

During operation, the pancreas can be approached through:

1. The gastrocolic ligament below the gastroepiploic arch (lesser sac)
2. The transverse mesocolon in the avascular area to the left of the middle colic vessels
3. The gastrohepatic ligament

A

ACID SUPPRESSION

Acid suppression (with H_2 receptor antagonists [H_2RAs] and proton pump inhibitors [PPIs]) is done in almost all patients with acute pancreatitis (although without much evidence to support it).

ACS

See **Abdominal compartment syndrome**

ACUTE ABDOMEN

Acute pancreatitis should be considered as a differential diagnosis in patients with acute (upper) abdomen along with other common conditions such as acute cholecystitis, perforated peptic ulcer, acute hepatitis, acute gastritis, and amebic liver abscess. The main aim of initial workup and investigations is to decide whether it is a surgical (e.g., peptic ulcer perforation) or a nonsurgical (e.g., acute pancreatitis) acute abdomen.

ACUTE CHOLECYSTITIS

Pain and vomiting in acute cholecystitis may mimic acute pancreatitis, with mild jaundice being present in both; guarding and tenderness in the right hypochondrium and Murphy's sign clinch the diagnosis. At a later stage (after a few days), a tender ill-defined inflammatory lump may be palpable in the right hypochondrium.

Leucocytosis is present and C-reactive protein is elevated in both conditions. Liver function tests (LFT) may show mild derangements. US is the investigation of choice; it shows gallstones, thick gallbladder wall (>3 mm) with pericholecystic edema, and fluid collection; pressure with the US probe elicits tenderness (sonographic Murphy's sign). CT shows the same findings as US with pericholecystic fat stranding. Isotope hepatobiliary scan shows nonvisualization of the gall bladder; if the gall bladder is seen on isotope scan, the diagnosis of acute cholecystitis is virtually ruled out. An attack of acute cholecystitis may be managed conservatively followed by elective cholecystectomy

4–6 weeks later. Alternatively, an early cholecystectomy may be performed, preferably within 3–5 days of onset of the attack.

A

ACUTE NECROTIC COLLECTION (ANC)

Early, nonwalled collection of solid debris (some fluid may also be present in addition) in and around the pancreas in acute necrotizing pancreatitis. It may be sterile or infected. ANC may either resolve or evolve into a WON.

ACUTE-ON-CHRONIC PANCREATITIS

Some attacks of acute pancreatitis occur on a background of chronic pancreatitis (Figure A.4) which can be clinically silent and may remain undiagnosed.

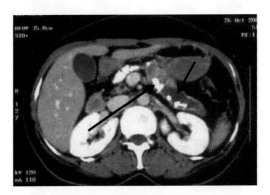

Figure A.4 Dilated pancreatic duct (small arrow) and calculi (large arrow) in **chronic pancreatitis**—an attack of acute pancreatitis can supervene.

ACUTE PANCREATITIS

Acute pancreatitis is defined as an acute inflammatory process of the pancreas with variable involvement of the regional tissues or remote organs. It could be acute interstitial (edematous) pancreatitis or acute necrotizing pancreatitis.

A ACUTE PERIPANCREATIC FLUID COLLECTION (APFC)

Early, nonwalled, ill-defined (confined by fascial planes) peripancreatic collection of fluid with no solid component (Figure A.5) in acute interstitial (edematous) pancreatitis.

Most APFCs resolve over 2–4 weeks; less than 10% persist beyond 4 weeks, develop a well-defined wall, and form a PPC (Figures A.6 and A.7).

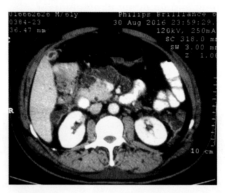

Figure A.5 Acute peripancreatic fluid collection.

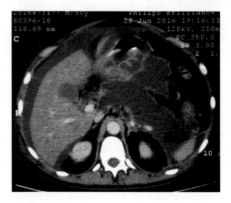

Figure A.6 Acute peripancreatic fluid collection in a patient (June 28, 2016).

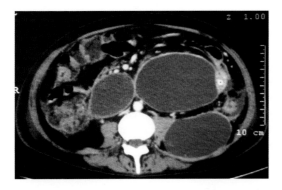

A

Figure A.7 Pseudocysts in the same patient one month later (July 28, 2016).

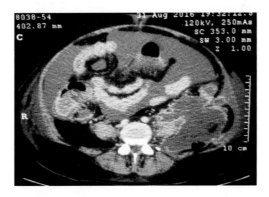

Figure A.8 Acute peripancreatic fluid collection not localized even 48 days after onset of acute pancreatitis.

In some patients, however, the fluid collection may not localize even after a long time (Figure A.8).

ADJACENT ORGANS

The inflammatory and necrotic process of acute pancreatitis may affect and involve adjacent organs (e.g., stomach, duodenum, proximal jejunum, transverse colon, and bile duct) and

A

adjacent vessels (e.g., splenic and middle colic arteries and portal vein).

ADMISSION

Based on the presence of various **risk factors** that predict **severity** of the attack, development of **local complications** and **organ dysfunction**, outcome, and mortality, patients with acute pancreatitis should be admitted to the general ward, HDU, or ICU.

AFFERENT LOOP OBSTRUCTION

Afferent loop obstruction after distal gastrectomy may cause acute pancreatitis.

AGE

Older (age >70 years) patients are more likely to have **severe** acute pancreatitis; they should preferably be managed in HDU/ICU.

AGGRESSIVE HYDRATION

Patients with acute pancreatitis have major fluid shifts and should be aggressively hydrated—up to 3–4 liters/day may be required to achieve urine output of at least 0.5 ml/Kg/hour.

AIR

Presence of air in necrosis (Figures A.9 and A.10) indicates infection or communication with bowel (usually transverse colon or proximal jejunum)—both being indications for intervention (percutaneous or surgical). Air may be present because of previous intervention, e.g., fine-needle aspiration (FNA), PCD, and surgery.

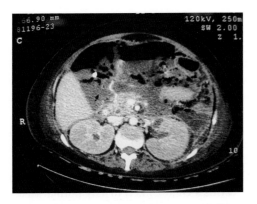

Figure A.9 Air in peripancreatic necrosis.

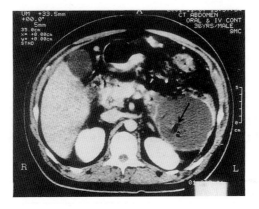

Figure A.10 Air in walled-off necrosis.

ALBUMIN

Intravenous albumin may be of use in increasing the osmotic pressure in hemodynamically unstable patients and in decreasing tissue edema. It, however, is not a nutritional supplement because of its short half-life.

A

ALCOHOL

Alcohol (along with gallstones) is an important, common, and preventable cause of acute pancreatitis. Acute pancreatitis occurs in those with a long (>3–5 years) history of intake of a large amount (about 100 g daily) of alcohol but may also occur in those with less intake. Alcohol alters pancreatic exocrine secretion, which results in the formation of precipitates in the pancreatic ducts causing obstruction and inflammation. Sometimes, a large dose of alcohol can precipitate an attack of acute pancreatitis. Alcohol also causes chronic pancreatitis. Patients with alcoholic acute pancreatitis are more likely to have normal serum **amylase**.

ALEXANDER

Alexander the Great of Macedon (Greece), who came all the way to the borders of India in 326 BC, is believed to have succumbed to alcoholic acute pancreatitis.

ALT (ALANINE TRANSAMINASE)

Elevated (>3 times normal) ALT (earlier called SGPT) levels within 48 hours in acute pancreatitis strongly suggest biliary etiology of acute pancreatitis.

AMBROSE PARE

Ambrose Pare of France first described acute pancreatitis in 1579.

AMI (ACUTE MESENTERIC ISCHEMIA)

AMI includes mesenteric vascular occlusion, e.g., mesenteric arterial embolism, mesenteric arterial or venous thrombosis, and nonocclusive mesenteric ischemia (NOMI).

AMI is a rare but serious cause of acute abdomen. Presentation is with sudden onset severe diffuse (ill localized) central (periumbilical) abdominal pain and can mimic acute pancreatitis. AMI should be suspected as the cause of an acute abdomen in patients with cardiac arrhythmias, e.g., atrial fibrillation and those with rheumatic valvular heart disease and those who have had a recent myocardial infarction (MI).

Serum **amylase** levels are elevated in AMI also, thus making it difficult to differentiate it from acute pancreatitis. A high index of suspicion and low threshold for investigation with contrast-enhanced CT and CT angiography can help in early diagnosis.

Early diagnosis of AMI is difficult; majority of the cases are diagnosed late when infarction, necrosis, and gangrene of the bowel and perforation and peritonitis have set in and need urgent surgical intervention.

AMINO ACIDS

Intravenous amino acids form an important component of parenteral nutrition and are safe in acute pancreatitis.

AMYLASE

Serum amylase is elevated (>3 times normal) in majority of patients with acute pancreatitis, but it is possible to have normal serum amylase level in acute pancreatitis (about 10% cases). Serum amylase levels increase soon (within hours) after the onset of acute pancreatitis; they peak in 48 hours and then settle in 3–5 days. Serum amylase has a low specificity for the diagnosis of acute pancreatitis and may be elevated in several other conditions such as acute cholecystitis, bowel ischemia gangrene and perforation, bowel obstruction, and gastroenteritis—all conditions that can mimic acute pancreatitis clinically. Serum amylase can be fractionated into pancreatic- and salivary-type isoamylases. Elevation of both serum amylase and **lipase** in a patient with **acute abdomen** is almost diagnostic of acute pancreatitis.

ANALGESIA

All patients with acute pancreatitis have severe **pain** and should receive adequate (parenteral) analgesia. Drugs such as morphine, pethidine, and pentazocine cause contraction of the sphincter of

A

Oddi and should be avoided. Diclofenac and tramadol may be used. Fentanyl drip and epidural analgesia are also useful.

See also **PCA**.

ANATOMIC ANOMALIES

Anatomic anomalies, e.g., **pancreas divisum**, long (>15 mm) **common channel** (of the common bile duct [CBD] and the pancreatic duct), may cause recurrent acute pancreatitis. These anomalies can be detected by ERCP or MRCP.

ANATOMY

The head of the pancreas occupies the concavity of the duodenal C loop. Uncinate process is an extension from the lower part of the head, projecting upward and to the left. The superior mesenteric vessels—vein and artery—lie on the surface of the uncinate process at the neck of the pancreas. The body of the pancreas is the main horizontal part extending across the midline in a slightly upward direction. The body is triangular in cross-section having anterior, superior, and inferior borders and antero-superior, antero-inferior, and posterior surfaces. Splenic artery runs along the superior border of the body of the pancreas while the splenic vein lies on its posterior surface. Transverse mesocolon originates at the anterior border of the body of the pancreas. The neck of the pancreas and its posterior surface are related to the junction of the superior mesenteric and splenic veins to form the portal vein and the origin of the superior mesenteric artery from the aorta. The portal vein can be easily separated from the posterior surface of the pancreas except in the presence of chronic inflammatory fibrosis and neoplastic infiltration. The tail of the pancreas lies in the lienorenal ligament and rests on the hilum of the spleen. The lower end of the CBD lies in a groove on the posterior surface of the head of the pancreas. CBD and the main pancreatic duct (of **Wirsung**) unite to form the ampulla of **Vater** which opens at the greater duodenal papilla surrounded by the sphincter of **Oddi**. The accessory pancreatic duct (of **Santorini**), which drains the upper part of the head of the pancreas, opens at the lesser duodenal papilla situated above the greater papilla.

ANGIOEMBOLIZATION

Radiological intervention in the form of angioembolization is the treatment of choice for a **pseudoaneurysm**. Steel or platinum coils, gelfoam, cyanoacrylate, or polyvinyl are substances used for embolization.

ANGIOGRAPHY

Conventional angiography (Figure A.11) is required for **embolization** of a **pseudoaneurysm** after it has been detected by noninvasive investigations such as **Doppler** US/endoscopic ultrasonography (EUS) or by CT angiography/MR angiography.

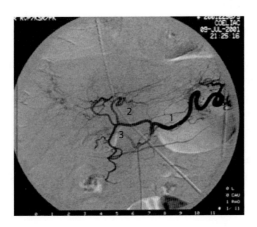

Figure A.11 Conventional **angiography** of the celiac axis showing (1) splenic, (2) common hepatic, and (3) gastroduodenal arteries.

ANNULAR PANCREAS

Annular pancreas is the second most common congenital anomaly (following pancreas divisum) of the pancreas. A ring of pancreatic

A

tissue encircles the second part of the duodenum. Severe cases may present as hydramnios in the mother. It may present as neonatal gastric outlet obstruction (double bubble on X-ray); less severe cases present in adulthood while mild cases remain asymptomatic. MRCP shows pancreatic duct around the CBD/duodenum. Annular pancreas does NOT cause acute pancreatitis.

ANOREXIA

Majority of patients with acute pancreatitis have anorexia and nausea; some may vomit also. This is because of gastroparesis caused by retrogastric/retroperitoneal inflammation. Oral intake is, therefore, poor and feeds should be given via nasogastric or nasojejunal tubes.

ANTIBIOTICS

Use of antibiotics in patients with acute pancreatitis is a debatable and contentious issue. Antibiotics are not indicated in patients with mild acute pancreatitis (even if they have fever and raised TLC/WBC counts). Most centers use antibiotics in patients with severe acute pancreatitis to prevent infection of necrosis which is the most important risk factor for mortality. Broad spectrum antibiotics should be used. Those with high pancreatic penetration (e.g., **fluoroquinolones** and **carbapenems**) are preferred. They should be administered intravenously. Prolonged use of antibiotics may, however, lead to emergence of resistant bacteria and opportunistic Gram-positive and **fungal** infections.

ANTIFUNGALS

Patients with severe acute pancreatitis are prone to fungal super-infection which increases mortality. Some centers use antifungal prophylaxis with **fluconazole** in patients with severe acute pancreatitis. In case of established fungal infection, therapeutic antifungals, e.g., polyenes (amphotericin), triazoles (voriconazole), and echinocandins (anidulafungin, caspofungin, micafungin), may be required.

ANTIOXIDANTS

Antioxidants have not been of any benefit in the treatment of acute pancreatitis.

AORTIC DISSECTION

Aortic dissection presents as sudden onset severe sharp stabbing or tearing chest or abdomen (or back) pain and may mimic acute pancreatitis. It is frequently seen in uncontrolled hypertensives. Discrepancy may be noted between the pulses of the right and left arms and legs. Suspicion of an abdominal aortic catastrophe (leaking or ruptured AAA or aortic dissection) is one of the indications for early, i.e., at the time of admission, contrast-enhanced CT in acute pancreatitis.

Transesophageal ECHO, CT, and MRI (of the chest and abdomen) are investigations of choice. Treatment includes rapid control of blood pressure (to stop further extension of the dissection) and surgical intervention.

APACHE (ACUTE PHYSIOLOGICAL AND CHRONIC HEALTH EVALUATION) II

APACHE uses 12 variables related to acute physiology score + age points + chronic health points. APACHE score is not specific to acute pancreatitis and can be used for any acute illness. Score ≥ 8 indicates severity of acute pancreatitis. High APACHE score is a risk factor for mortality as well. The advantage of APACHE over **Ranson** score is that it can be obtained at admission without waiting for 48 hours. Main disadvantage is that it is very cumbersome to obtain.

APACHE O

APACHE O includes **obesity** as a factor. Obesity is an independent risk factor for mortality in severe acute pancreatitis.

A

APPROACH

Pancreas can be approached through gastrocolic (wider access to lesser sac), infra mesocolic (if gastrocolic approach is difficult), and gastrohepatic and paracolic routes.

APROTININ

Aprotinin, a **trypsin** inhibitor, has not been shown to have any useful effect on the course and outcome of acute pancreatitis and is not recommended for use.

ARDS (ADULT RESPIRATORY DISTRESS SYNDROME)

ARDS may be present in patients with severe acute pancreatitis as a part of MODS. ARDS is characterized by tachypnea, rhonchi, crepitations, and bilateral hilar fluffy infiltrates on chest X-ray. SpO_2 remains low in spite of high FiO_2. Treatment is positive end-expiratory pressure (PEEP) ventilation.

ARF (ACUTE RENAL FAILURE)

ARF can occur in patients with severe acute pancreatitis as a part of MODS. Contrast used during CT or angiography and nephrotoxic drugs (e.g., some antibiotics and analgesics) may also contribute. ARF is a strong predictor of mortality in acute pancreatitis. ARF should be prevented in patients with acute pancreatitis by adequate hydration, maintenance of normotension, and avoidance of nephrotoxic drugs, including IV contrast used in CT and MRI.

ASCARIASIS

In areas where it is common (e.g., in Kashmir), infestation of the biliary tract with roundworm (*Ascaris lumbricoides*) can cause acute pancreatitis.

ASCITES, PANCREATIC

Pancreatic ascites is caused by disruption of the pancreatic duct or leak/rupture of a **pseudocyst** into the peritoneal cavity. It is more common in patients with acute-on-chronic pancreatitis; it may occur following pancreatic **trauma** (Figure A.12a and A.12b) also.

Ascitic fluid has high protein (>3 g/dL) and **amylase** (>100,000 U/L) levels. Initial management is conservative and includes nil by mouth, nasogastric aspiration and drainage,

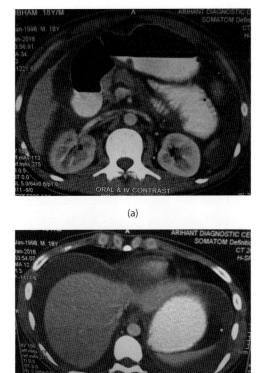

(a)

(b)

Figure A.12 (a) Traumatic fracture of the neck of the pancreas causing (b) pancreatic ascites.

A

total parenteral nutrition (TPN), and **octreotide**. Paracentesis may be required in some cases. Persistent pancreatic ascites in spite of conservative management for 2–4 weeks needs intervention. Endoscopic intervention includes pancreatic sphincterotomy and placement of a stent in the pancreatic duct across the site of leak. Surgical treatment includes anastomosis of a Roux-en-Y loop of jejunum to the pancreatic duct or the pseudocyst.

ASPIRATION

It is recommended to aspirate peripancreatic **necrosis** (under US or CT guidance) for Gram staining and culture to rule out/diagnose **infection**.

ATELECTASIS

Patients with acute pancreatitis may have atelectasis (Figure A.13), pneumonitis, and pleural effusion—usually at the base on the left side.

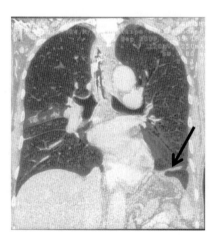

Figure A.13 Basal **atelectasis** (left) in acute pancreatitis.

ATLANTA CLASSIFICATION

A

An international symposium on acute pancreatitis held in 1992 at Atlanta, GA, USA, defined acute pancreatitis as an acute inflammatory process of the pancreas with variable involvement of regional and remote organs (Bradley 1993). Acute pancreatitis was classified into mild and severe based on clinical and investigative parameters. **Severe** acute pancreatitis was defined as acute pancreatitis with **organ failure** and/or local complications, e.g., **necrosis, pseudocyst,** or **abscess.**

The original Atlanta classification was not accepted and utilized universally as it was found that it had several shortcomings.

The revised Atlanta classification (2012) introduced another level of severity—moderate acute pancreatitis (Sarr et al. 2013). Local complications were reclassified as APFC, PPC, ANC, and WON; the term "pancreatic **abscess**" was dropped.

ATLANTA CRITERIA

For severe acute pancreatitis

1. **Organ failure**
   Shock—systolic BP <90 mm
   Pulmonary insufficiency PaO_2 <60 mm Hg Renal failure—serum creatinine >2 mg/dL gastrointestinal bleeding >500 ml/24 hours
2. Local complications, e.g., **pseudocyst, necrosis,** and **abscess**

The revised (2012) modification of Atlanta Criteria has defined severe pancreatitis as persistent organ failure.

AUTOIMMUNE PANCREATITIS (AIP)

Patients with AIP present with pain and weight loss; imaging shows a sausage-shaped 'mass' in pancreas (Figure A.14) and pancreaticogram (ERP or MRP) reveals diffusely irregular pancreatic duct. Differential diagnosis from pancreatic cancer and chronic

A

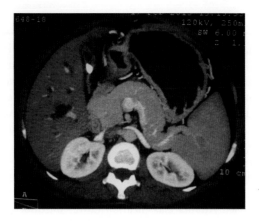

Figure A.14 CT showing sausage-shaped enlargement of the pancreas in autoimmune pancreatitis.

pancreatitis is, therefore, difficult. Attacks of acute pancreatitis may occur but are rare. Multiple organs (e.g., liver and kidney) may be involved. Serum IgG is elevated, and antibodies, e.g., anti-nuclear antibody (ANA), are present. Treatment is with steroids but many patients undergo resection as malignancy cannot be excluded.

B

BACTERIA

The most frequent organisms isolated from infected necrosis in patients with severe acute necrotizing pancreatitis are of enteric origin, i.e., *Escherichia coli, Klebsiella pneumoniae,* and *enterococci.*

BALTHAZAR

CT severity index (CTSI) of Balthazar includes:

1. Grade of acute pancreatitis
   a. normal pancreas (0)
   b. focal or diffuse enlargement of pancreas with irregularity or heterogeneous enhancement (1)
   c. inflammation confined to pancreas/peripancreatic fat (2)
   d. one peripancreatic fluid collection (3)
   e. two or more peripancreatic fluid collections or gas (4)
2. Degree of pancreatic necrosis
   a. Nil (0)
   b. One-third of the gland (2)
   c. One-half of the gland (4)
   d. More than half of the gland (6)

   CTSI = Grade of acute pancreatitis + degree of necrosis
          (maximum of 10)

CTSI	Complications (%)	Mortality (%)
0–3	8	3
4–6	35	6
7–10	92	15–20

BARRIER, GUT MUCOSAL

The disruption of gut mucosal barrier because of inflammation is one of the important mechanisms for **infection** of **necrosis** due to **translocation** of bacteria across the gut wall in severe acute pancreatitis.

BASE DEFICIT

Base deficit (and low **pH**) in arterial blood gas (ABG) is a marker for poor outcome in acute pancreatitis.

BEGER

Hans G. Beger of Ulm, Germany, advocated **closed drainage** and continuous **lavage** after **necrosectomy**.

BIMODAL

Severe acute pancreatitis has a bimodal pattern of mortality—early (within 2 weeks of onset) deaths due to multiple organ failure (MOF) as a result of systemic inflammatory response syndrome (SIRS) and late (after 4 weeks of onset) deaths due to septic complications of **infected necrosis**.

BINGE

A binge of alcohol may often precipitate an attack of acute pancreatitis.

BIOLOGICAL MARKERS

Various biological markers, e.g., C-reactive protein (CRP), trypsinogen-activation peptide (TAP), interleukin (IL)-6, and procalcitonin (PCT), are elevated in acute pancreatitis. Their estimation is not essential for clinical management of acute pancreatitis; they are mainly of academic/research interest.

BIOPSY

During surgical drainage of a **pseudocyst**, a disc of the cyst wall is excised (Figure B.1) to obtain a larger stoma; also, the excised disc of the cyst wall should be sent for histopathological examination to rule out a **cystic neoplasm** of the pancreas for which complete excision (and NOT internal drainage, as is done for a pseudocyst) is the appropriate management. Presence of an epithelial lining in the cyst wall suggests the diagnosis of a true cyst or cystic neoplasm as pseudocyst wall has no epithelial lining.

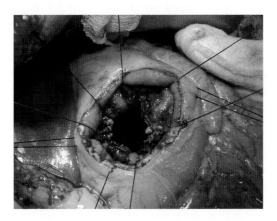

Figure B.1 Disc of the posterior wall of the stomach and the anterior wall of the pseudocyst being excised for **biopsy** during cystogastrostomy.

BIPAP

Biphasic positive airway pressure ventilation—a noninvasive method of ventilation used while weaning a patient from invasive ventilation.

BISAP SCORE

Bedside index for severity of acute pancreatitis (BISAP)—age >60 years, impaired mental status, SIRS, BUN >25 mg, and

B

pleural effusion indicate severity and poor outcome in acute pancreatitis.

BLEED

1. Spontaneous bleed may occur in a preexisting **pseudocyst** (Figure B.2a and B.2b) due to erosion into an adjacent vessel, e.g., splenic, gastroduodenal, middle colic, and left gastric artery. It is also a complication of percutaneous, endoscopic, or surgical drainage of a pseudocyst.

   Angiographic **embolization** is the treatment of choice; if it fails, emergency surgery has to be performed to doubly ligate or suture ligate the bleeding artery, although this is technically very difficult and demanding.

   Gastrointestinal (GI) bleed can be caused by erosive mucosal disease (EMD) or gastric varices caused due to splenic vein thrombosis (SVT).

   Intraperitoneal/retroperitoneal bleed (Figures B.3 and B.4) can be caused by enzymatic destruction of peripancreatic vessels (arteries and veins) in pancreatic necrosis (Figure B.5).

   Bleeding is associated with high mortality, still higher if an associated **fistula** is present.
2. Bleeding during necrosectomy indicates that dissection has reached normal viable tissue and should stop.

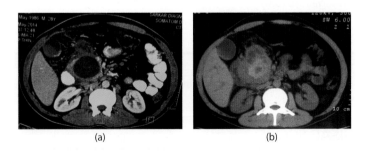

(a)   (b)

Figure B.2 (a) Intrapancreatic pseudocyst on May 1, 2014 and (b) intracystic **bleed** (enhanced) on June 11, 2014.

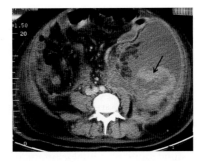

Figure B.3 **Bleed** (seen as enhancing area on IV contrast CT) in necrosis.

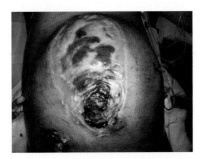

Figure B.4 Major extraperitoneal **bleed** in pancreatic necrosis.

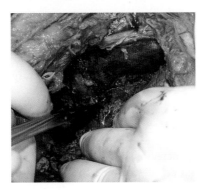

Figure B.5 Necrotic vessel in pancreatic necrosis—the vessel can give way and cause massive fatal **bleed**.

BLEEDING, GASTROINTESTINAL

B

Patients with acute pancreatitis may have gastrointestinal (GI) bleed due to several reasons:

1. Portal hypertension and esophagogastric varices due to splenic vein **thrombosis**; treatment is endoscopic (variceal band ligation, glue injection, or sclerotherapy)
2. A **pseudoaneurysm** rupturing into an adjacent viscus, e.g., stomach, duodenum, proximal jejunum, or colon; treatment is angioembolization
3. Erosion of a **pseudocyst** into stomach, duodenum, jejunum, or colon; bleed may settle with treatment of the pseudocyst

BLEEDING, INTRAOPERATIVE

Necrosectomy, if performed early, when the necrotic process has not been well localized and demarcation between necrotic and viable tissue is not clear, may be associated with excessive bleeding. This usually needs packing and reoperation after 24–48 hours for pack removal.

Bleeding can also occur as a result of adjacent vessels, e.g., gastroduodenal, splenic, middle colic, and left gastric, giving way due to inflammatory necrosis of the wall of the vessel.

BLEEDING, RETROPERITONEAL

Pancreatic necrosis can erode into retroperitoneal vessels to cause a large hematoma—if significant, it requires surgical evacuation and packing.

BLOOD SUPPLY

The head of the pancreas is supplied by anterior and posterior pancreaticoduodenal arcades formed by the anterior and posterior superior pancreaticoduodenal arteries from the gastroduodenal artery and anterior and posterior inferior pancreaticoduodenal arteries from the superior mesenteric artery. The body of the pancreas receives its blood supply from the splenic artery via transverse pancreatic, superior pancreatic, posterior pancreatic, and greater pancreatic branches. Caudal pancreatic arteries (also from the splenic artery) supply the tail.

Head and neck of the pancreas are drained by anterior and posterior pancreaticoduodenal veins which drain into the portal vein. A branch of the anterior pancreaticoduodenal venous arcade joins the right gastroepiploic vein to form the gastrocolic vein draining into the superior mesenteric vein. **Veins** draining the body and the tail directly join the splenic vein.

BMI (BODY MASS INDEX)

$$BMI = Weight\ (Kg)/Height\ (m)^2$$

Obesity with BMI >30 predicts poor outcome in **severe** acute pancreatitis.

BOGGY

Necrosis has a characteristic soft boggy putty-like feel. This differentiates it from normal (viable) surrounding tissue, which feels soft to firm, during **necrosectomy**. **Finger** is the best instrument to differentiate between necrotic and viable tissues.

BOWEL

Bowel, in acute pancreatitis, is inflamed, edematous, and friable; it should be handled very gently to avoid an iatrogenic perforation. For the same reason, a bowel anastomosis should be avoided in the presence of acute pancreatitis.

BOWEL REST

In the first few days of acute pancreatitis, bowel should be rested—nil by mouth (NBM).

BRADLEY

Edward L. Bradley, III of Emory University, Atlanta, GA, USA, advocated **open packing** (**laparostomy**) after **necrosectomy**.

BRONCHOSCOPY

Bronchoscopic toilet may help in removing secretions and mucous plugs in the collapsed segments of lungs in patients with severe acute pancreatitis.

BUY TIME

In patients in the early phase (1st–3rd week) of acute pancreatitis, percutaneous intervention (needle aspiration or catheter drainage of the peripancreatic fluid collection) may buy time by controlling infection and delaying surgical intervention to an appropriate late phase (4th week) of the illness.

C

CALCIUM

Normal total serum calcium level is 2.2–2.6 mmol/L (9.0–10.5 mg/dL)

1. **Hypercalcaemia** can cause recurrent acute pancreatitis.
2. Patients with severe acute pancreatitis may develop **hypocalcaemia** and require IV administration of calcium gluconate.

CALORIES

Patients with severe acute pancreatitis are in **catabolism**—they should receive a high (25–30 nonprotein Kcal/kg or about 2000–3000 Kcal/day) high-protein diet. In case of SIRS or MODS, this can be reduced to 15–20 Kcal/Kg.

CAN (CONTRAST-ASSOCIATED NEPHROPATHY)

IV contrast used during CT is nephrotoxic. Nonionic contrast media are associated with less risk of CAN and should be used in patients with acute pancreatitis. N-acetyl-L-cysteine (NAC) prior to CT may reduce the risk of CAN.

CANCER

A small pancreatic/periampullary cancer may present as acute pancreatitis.

Endoscopic ultrasonography (EUS) is a good investigation to detect a small mass lesion.

CANDIDA

Prolonged use of broad spectrum **antibiotics** predisposes patients with severe acute pancreatitis to **fungal** infections. Prophylactic use of antifungal **fluconazole** may reduce the incidence of Candida infection; this is, however, not a universal clinical practice.

CARBAPENEMS

Carbapenems, e.g., imipenem, meropenem, and doripenem, are **antibiotics** of choice for patients with severe acute pancreatitis as they have good penetration in pancreas and have a broad spectrum of cover against Gram-positive and Gram-negative aerobes as well as anaerobes.

CARS

Compensatory anti-inflammatory syndrome (another name for SIRS).

CATABOLISM

Patients with severe acute pancreatitis are in severe catabolism, akin to those with systemic sepsis, extensive burns, and polytrauma, and have very high energy and protein requirements.

CAUSES

See **Etiology**

CBD EVALUATION

In patients with biliary acute pancreatitis, common bile duct (CBD) is evaluated with liver function tests (LFTs) and ultrasonography (US). Patients with a CBD stone on US should undergo endoscopic retrograde cholangiography (ERC) and therapeutic intervention. Those with dilated CBD or deranged LFT should have their CBD evaluated by magnetic resonance cholangiography (MRC)—only those found to have CBD stone on MRC should have ERC. EUS is also useful for diagnosis of CBD stones.

CENTRAL

Acute pancreatitis usually presents as upper abdominal (epigastric) pain, but in some patients pain may be felt in the central abdomen (periumbilical).

C

CHALLENGE

Management of severe acute pancreatitis is a challenge for even an experienced physician/surgeon.

CHDF

Continuous hemodiafiltration (CHDF) may be of use to remove **cytokines** in patients with MODS (including renal dysfunction).

CHEST X-RAY

1. Chest X-ray, including both domes of diaphragm, must be obtained in all patients with acute pancreatitis. Presence of free air under the domes of diaphragm confirms a diagnosis of a perforated viscus—an important differential diagnosis of acute pancreatitis.
2. A large number of patients with acute pancreatitis will have left pleural effusion and basal **atelectasis**. Patients with severe acute pancreatitis and multiple organ dysfunction syndrome (MODS) may show changes of adult respiratory distress syndrome (ARDS) on chest X-ray.

CHOLANGIOGRAM

1. Patients with severe (biliary) acute pancreatitis should have an early (within 48–72 hours) endoscopic retrograde cholangiography (ERC) and endoscopic papillotomy (EPT) and stone extraction.
2. Patients undergoing interval cholecystectomy after an attack of acute pancreatitis can have common bile duct (CBD) evaluation with magnetic resonance cholangiography (MRC) or

endoscopic ultrasonography (EUS); endoscopic retrograde cholangiography (ERC) is indicated only if a CBD stone is found on MRC or EUS.

CHOLANGITIS

In patients with gallstone acute pancreatitis, uncontrolled cholangitis due to CBD stones (rather than severe acute pancreatitis itself) may be the indication for endoscopic intervention in the form of EPT/stenting.

CHOLECYSTECTOMY

In patients with biliary acute pancreatitis, cholecystectomy should be performed as soon as possible to prevent a recurrent attack of acute pancreatitis.

In patients with mild (gallstone) acute pancreatitis, cholecystectomy may be performed in the same hospital admission.

In patients with severe (gallstone) acute pancreatitis, cholecystectomy should be performed when inflammation has settled as evidenced by clinical picture and investigations (total leucocyte counts TLC, CRP, US/CT)—this is usually 4–6 weeks after the attack of acute pancreatitis has settled.

In a patient with walled-off necrosis (WON), cholecystectomy may be performed at the time of necrosectomy (Figure C.1)

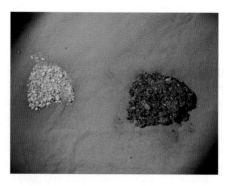

Figure C.1 Gallstones and necrotic debris.

if the patient is stable and if the right upper quadrant is easily accessible.

If for some reason, cholecystectomy cannot be performed as indicated above, an EPT (with or without placement of an endobiliary stent) may be considered.

C

CHOLEDOCHAL CYST

Patients with choledochal cyst may suffer from recurrent attacks of acute pancreatitis.

Choledochal cyst can be diagnosed on US/MRC (Figure C.2).

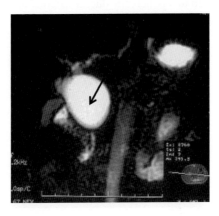

Figure C.2 MRCP showing **choledochal cyst**.

CHOLEDOCHOCELE

A choledochocele at the lower end of the CBD may cause acute pancreatitis due to obstruction of the pancreatic duct. It can be diagnosed on MRC/EUS.

CHOLESTEROL

Cholesterol crystals should be looked for in the duodenal bile in patients with recurrent acute pancreatitis if US does not reveal gallstones. Such patients may benefit from cholecystectomy.

CHRONIC PANCREATITIS

1. An attack of acute pancreatitis may occur superimposed on underlying chronic pancreatitis (CP) (which may or may not be known in a given patient). All patients with acute pancreatitis without a known common cause, e.g., gallstones, alcohol, and patients with **recurrent** acute pancreatitis should be investigated for CP. This is done by obtaining a pancreaticogram (MRP or ERP) which shows irregularity and dilatation of the pancreatic duct (Figure C.3).

2. Acute pancreatitis with disruption of the main pancreatic duct may lead to a pancreatic ductal stricture and downstream chronic pancreatitis with ductal dilatation.

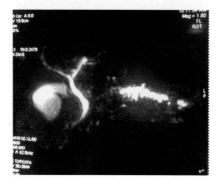

Figure C.3 This patient had recurrent attacks of acute pancreatitis; MRCP shows dilated irregular pancreatic duct suggestive of chronic pancreatitis.

CLINICAL PICTURE

Patients with acute pancreatitis present with sudden onset severe upper abdominal pain, nausea/vomiting, and fever.

CLOSED LAVAGE

After **necrosectomy**, lesser sac may be closed after two to four wide bore (28–32 F) drains are placed in it; **continuous lavage** follows.

CLOSED LAPAROSTOMA

Semiopen technique (cf. **closed drainage**, **laparostomy**, and open **packing**)—abdomen is closed not with suture but with a **zipper** or a sheet of prosthetic material (e.g., Mesh) sutured to its edges. This is associated with less fluid and electrolyte and protein loss when compared with open laparostomy.

COLECTOMY

Colectomy may rarely be required for a segment of ischemic or frankly gangrenous and perforated transverse colon adjacent to the inflamed pancreas. This should be followed by proximal fistula and distal mucus fistula; anastomosis must be avoided.

COLLECTION, FLUID

See **Fluid collection**

COLLOIDS

Too much colloids should be avoided during resuscitation as they have an adverse effect on lung function.

COLON

Because of its proximity to the pancreas (transverse), colon plays a very important role in acute pancreatitis. **Translocation** of luminal bacteria across the inflamed colonic wall results in **infection** of peripancreatic **fluid collections** and **necrosis**. Transverse colon may form part of the wall of a (peri) pancreatic **abscess**; ascending and descending colon may similarly be involved in infracolic inflammation/necrosis. Colonic involvement may manifest as lower GI **bleed**, necrosis of the wall, and **perforation** of colon. A prophylactic proximal **ileostomy** may be indicated in such cases. Some patients may even require **colectomy**.

C

COLONIC FISTULA

A colonic perforation/fistula secondary to bowel ischemia and gangrene in acute necrotizing pancreatitis may require a proximal diverting **ileostomy** or even segmental **colectomy** (with proximal stoma and distal mucus fistula).

COLON CUT OFF

Inflamed pancreas may cause edematous obstruction of the transverse colon—plain X-ray of abdomen shows dilated ascending and proximal transverse colon with no air beyond.

COLOSTOMY

Transverse colostomy is almost never possible in acute pancreatitis—colon is inflamed, edematous and thickened, and mesocolon is shortened; if proximal bowel diversion is required, an **ileostomy** should be performed.

COMBINATION

Combination of necrosis, infection, and organ failure has the worst prognosis in acute pancreatitis.

COMMENSALS

Commensals, e.g., Gram-positive cocci and fungi, become clinically important after prolonged use of broad spectrum **antibiotics** in patients with severe acute pancreatitis.

COMMON CHANNEL

In majority (85%) of cases, the pancreatic duct and the CBD unite to form a common channel which opens through a single opening at the tip of the papilla into the medial wall of the second part of the duodenum. The common channel, when dilated, is called ampulla (of **Vater**); a long (>15 mm) common channel predisposes to recurrent acute pancreatitis.

COMMUNICATION

1. A pseudocyst may communicate with the pancreatic duct—more often in chronic pancreatitis than in acute pancreatitis.
2. Patients with severe acute pancreatitis can be very sick and take a sudden turn for the worse—frequent and regular communication with the relatives about the condition of the patient and his/her progress will go to a great extent to avoid a medicolegal suit even in case of a mishap (mortality) in a patient with acute pancreatitis.

C

COMPLEX

Acute pancreatitis is one of the most complex acute abdominal conditions to diagnose, to manage, and even to prognosticate.

COMPLICATIONS

1. Local complications of acute pancreatitis include **fluid collection**; **pseudocyst**; GI **bleed**; biliary, duodenal, and colonic obstruction; vascular complications, e.g., arterial **pseudoaneurysm**; and splenic vein thrombosis (SVT). Persistence of abdominal pain, fever (with chills), secondary increase in serum enzymes (amylase/lipase), and development of organ failure should raise the suspicion of local complications.
2. Complications of surgical management of acute pancreatitis (necrosectomy) include bleeding from the necrotic cavity, necrosis of adjacent bowel (colon, jejunum), and enterocutaneous fistula and pancreatic fistula.

COMPLEMENTARY

Interventional radiology, therapeutic endoscopy, and surgical intervention complement each other in the overall management of a patient with severe acute pancreatitis.

CONSERVATIVE

It is safer to be conservative while doing **necrosectomy** so that the dissection does not enter viable tissues (in order to avoid **bleeding**)—this may result in some residual necrosis which may resolve on its own or may require reintervention. A "radical" necrosectomy may result in the dissection getting into viable tissues, resulting in profuse uncontrollable bleeding.

CONSERVATIVE MANAGEMENT

Conservative management of mild acute pancreatitis includes nil by mouth (NBM), nasogastric aspiration and drainage (if the patient is vomiting) and intravenous fluids. Antibiotics are not required. Majority of cases with mild acute pancreatitis will resolve with this treatment in 3–5 days.

Sterile necrosis and few patients with infected necrosis, who are stable, can be managed conservatively without **intervention**.

CONTINUOUS LAVAGE

After **closed drainage** of the lesser sac, continuous lavage is done with large (6–24 liters per day) volumes of saline/dialysis fluid. Lavage should continue till the returns are clear, sterile, and amylase free—this may take weeks, rather than days.

CORONARY BYPASS

Coronary bypass surgery can cause acute pancreatitis.

COSTS

Costs of management of a patient with severe acute pancreatitis may be very high due to prolonged hospitalization (including admission to the intensive care unit or ICU/high dependency unit or HDU), repeated investigations and interventions, expensive antibiotics, parenteral nutrition, etc. In some patients, it is not only the disease but also the cost of its management which kills the patient (and the family).

COUNSELING

1. Treatment of severe acute pancreatitis involves prolonged hospitalization, including ICU stay, repeated investigations and interventions, expensive medicines (antibiotics and parenteral nutrition), complications, ups and downs in the course of illness, and highly unpredictable outcome. At the same time, however, if the patient recovers, he or she may lead a near normal life. It is, therefore, very important to properly counsel the patient and the relatives about the management, prognosis, and outcome.
2. Patients with acute alcoholic pancreatitis should be counseled at the time of discharge from the hospital regarding the risks of recurrent disease and the benefits of abstinence.

CPAP

Continuous positive airway pressure ventilation—a noninvasive method of ventilation used during weaning from invasive ventilation. It prevents the alveoli from collapsing and keeps them open.

CRE

Controlled radial expansion (CRE) wire-guided balloon to dilate (up to 12–15 mm) the opening into the pseudocyst during its endoscopic drainage into the stomach.

CRITERIA

Several criteria, e.g., **Atlanta**, **Ranson's**, Glasgow (**Imrie**), and **Balthazar**, are used for scoring the severity of acute pancreatitis.

CRP (C-REACTIVE PROTEIN)

CRP, an acute-phase protein, is a nonspecific marker of inflammation and may be elevated in a patient with mild acute pancreatitis and associated inflammation in other organs, e.g., acute cholangitis due to associated CBD stones. CRP reaches its peak about 96 hours after the onset of acute pancreatitis. CRP >150 mg/L

(>300 mg/mL in some reports) indicates severe acute pancreatitis with 80%–90% sensitivity.

CRRT

Continuous renal replacement therapy (CRRT) is indicated in the presence of volume overload, hyperkalemia, metabolic **acidosis**, and progressive azotemia in patients with acute pancreatitis and acute renal failure (ARF).

CRYSTALS

In patients with **idiopathic** acute pancreatitis, duodenal bile should be obtained after cholecystokinin (CCK) stimulation and examined for cholesterol monohydrate or calcium bilirubinate crystals. Such patients may benefit from cholecystectomy.

CT (COMPUTED TOMOGRAPHY)

CT is not essential to make a diagnosis of acute pancreatitis, if clinical and biochemical picture is highly suggestive. It may be required in a few cases when the diagnosis is in doubt and a surgical cause, e.g., peptic ulcer perforation, acute mesenteric ischemia (AMI), leaking/ruptured abdominal aortic aneurysm (AAA) of **acute abdomen**, cannot be excluded.

All patients with acute pancreatitis do not need CT—those with mild acute pancreatitis do not need a CT if they are showing expected clinical improvement.

A good quality, thin (<5 mm) slice, multislice, contrast (100–150 mL IV contrast injected at a rate of 3 mL/sec) enhanced multidetector (MD) CT (Figure C.4) is the most important investigation for diagnosis of pancreatic **necrosis** which is seen as nonenhancing pancreatic parenchyma. CT is also useful for the assessment of severity, planning of management, and assessment of progress in acute pancreatitis. It should be obtained after 3–4 days of onset of acute pancreatitis as necrosis takes about 48–72 hours to develop and about 96 hours to fully establish (The author prefers to get CT done after about 5–7 days of onset of acute pancreatitis).

C

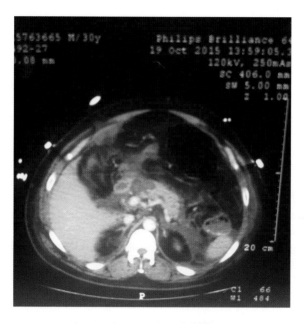

Figure C.4 Contrast-enhanced CT showing nonenhancing parenchyma (necrosis) in the neck; distal body, and tail are enhancing.

CT may have to be repeated to detect complications of acute pancreatitis, especially if the patient is not responding to treatment or is deteriorating. Suspicion of a postnecrosectomy complication is also an indication for CT.

Early (at admission) CT should be done if the diagnosis of acute pancreatitis is in doubt—mainly to rule out surgical conditions causing **acute abdomen**, e.g., perforation—peritonitis, AMI, leaking/ruptured AAA, etc., or if there is suspicion of a **local complication**, e.g., **bleeding** or **perforation**, which may require intervention.

Patient should be resuscitated and well hydrated and renal functions evaluated before a CT is done as the IV contrast is nephrotoxic and can cause CAN. Pancreatic inflammation—diffuse homogenous edematous enlargement of the gland, with blurred irregular outline, peripancreatic fat stranding, anterior perinephric

(**Gerota's**) fascial thickening, and peripancreatic fluid collection; ascites; and pleural effusion (usually left) suggest acute pancreatitis, but a normal pancreas on CT does not rule out acute pancreatitis as CT may be normal in a patient with mild acute pancreatitis.

CT should be obtained in patients with **pseudocyst** just before intervention to delineate the site (location), especially in relation to stomach/duodenum; size and number of the pseudocysts; wall thickness (one may have to wait for intervention if the wall is not mature); contents (all fluid when percutaneous/endoscopic intervention is more likely to be successful versus lot of solid debris when surgical intervention is better); presence of any enhancing **pseudoaneurysm** (Figure C.5), which should be angioembolized before any intervention on the cyst; and presence of any biliary obstruction (in case of a cyst near the head of the pancreas).

Threshold for asking for a CT in acute necrotizing pancreatitis should be low. In young patients, however, the risk of excessive radiation exposure should be kept in mind if multiple CTs are required; MRI is preferred over CT.

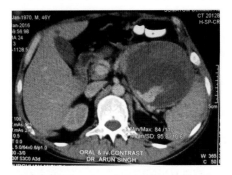

Figure C.5 CT showing an enhancing lesion within a pseudocyst.

CT ATTENUATION

CT attenuation value of normal pancreas is about 40–50 Hounsfield Units (HU) on nonenhanced scan and about 100–150 HU on an enhanced scan. Nonenhanced pancreatic parenchyma on contrast-enhanced CT suggests **necrosis**.

CTSI (CT SEVERITY INDEX)

CT severity index of **Balthazar** is a useful predictor of outcome and mortality

$$CTSI = CT\ grade + necrosis\ index$$

Modified CTSI includes extrapancreatic complications also.

CULLEN'S SIGN

Bluish discoloration around the umbilicus in acute pancreatitis—*rarely seen in clinical practice.*

CVC

Central venous catheter (CVC) will be inserted in virtually all patients with severe acute pancreatitis either for monitoring of central venous pressure (CVP) or for administration of parenteral nutrition. CVCs may be associated with several complications, e.g., bleeding, pneumothorax, catheter-related infections (CRI), and blood stream infections (BSI).

CVVHD

Continuous venovenous hemodiafiltration (CVVHD) as an alternative to hemodialysis in patients with ARF as part of MODS.

CYANOSIS

Patients with severe acute pancreatitis and MODS may have cyanosis due to **hypoxia** caused by respiratory failure.

CYST

A true pancreatic cyst is lined with epithelium (cf. **pseudocyst** which has a wall of inflammatory granulation and fibrous tissue without an epithelial lining). A true cyst needs excision (cf. drainage for pseudocyst).

CYSTIC FIBROSIS

Patients with cystic fibrosis (mucoviscidosis) due to cystic fibrosis transmembrane (CFTR) gene mutation are more prone to have recurrent acute pancreatitis.

CYSTIC NEOPLASM

The possibility that a **pseudocyst** (Figure C.6) may be a cystic neoplasm (Figure C.7), e.g., mucinous cystic neoplasm (MCN)

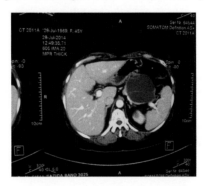

Figure C.6 Misdiagnosed initially as a pseudocyst, this finally turned out to be a mucinous cystic neoplasm.

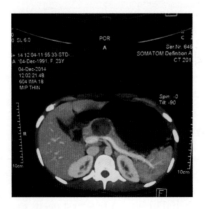

Figure C.7 **Cystic neoplasm** in tail of pancreas.

or intraductal papillary mucinous neoplasm (IPMN), should be kept in mind. Cyst fluid may be obtained by US-/CT-/EUS-guided needle aspiration for cytology, **amylase**, and tumor marker (CEA) estimation. A disc of the cyst wall must be excised and sent for histopathology when draining a pseudocyst.

CYSTODUODENOSTOMY

A **pseudocyst** near the head of the pancreas may be drained into the duodenum. The site of drainage in the duodenum should be carefully selected to avoid injury to the CBD.

CYSTOGASTROSTOMY

A **pseudocyst** which projects into the posterior wall of the stomach is best drained into the stomach by cystogastrostomy (Figure C.8). Bleeding from the stomach wall is a common complication of cystogastrostomy; an interlocking continuous hemostatic suture should, therefore, be used.

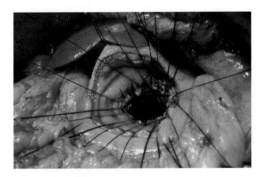

Figure C.8 **Cystogastrostomy** in progress.

Cystogastrostomy can be performed endoscopically also if the cyst is in approximation with the posterior wall of the stomach and its contents are mainly fluid (Figures C9a and C9b).

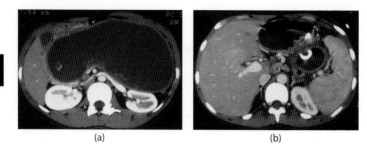

Figure C.9 (a) A large pseudocyst behind the stomach with mainly fluid contents and (b) after endoscopic cystogastrostomy (stent is in situ).

CYSTOJEJUNOSTOMY

A **pseudocyst** so located that it cannot be drained into the stomach or the duodenum is drained into a Roux-en-Y loop of jejunum.

Large pseudocysts which are projecting mainly below the transverse mesocolon and those mainly in the head/tail of the pancreas are not suited for **cystogastrostomy** and are better managed by cystojejunostomy.

Some surgeons, as a matter of choice, drain all pseudocysts, irrespective of their location, into the jejunum.

CYTOKINE STORM

Sudden release of proinflammatory mediators (cytokines), e.g., interleukins (IL), platelet-activating factor (PAF), and tumor necrosis factor (TNF), by the macrophages into the blood stream is responsible for producing SIRS in the early stages of acute pancreatitis.

D

DEBRIDEMENT

A term, although incorrect, used for **necrosectomy**, usually followed by packing.

DEBRIS

A small amount of debris (Figure D.1) may be present in a **pancreatic pseudocyst** (which is mainly a collection of fluid). CT is not a good investigation to detect solid debris; it is better seen on ultrasonography (US) or MRI.

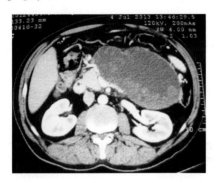

Figure D.1 CT showing significant amount of solid necrotic debris in a pseudocyst.

DECONTAMINATION, SELECTIVE GUT

See **Selective gut decontamination**

DEFICIENCY

Severe acute pancreatitis, especially after **necrosectomy**, may result in endocrine (diabetes) and exocrine (steatorrhea) deficiency.

DEFINITION

Acute pancreatitis is defined as an acute inflammatory process of the pancreas, with variable involvement of regional tissues and remote organs, with eventual clinical, biochemical, and radiological reversal of the inflammation.

DELAY

Management of acute pancreatitis in the early phase (1st–3rd week) is largely conservative/nonsurgical (unless there is **bleeding, gangrene**, or **perforation**). If intervention is required in the early phase for drainage of infected fluid collections, it should preferably be done percutaneously. Surgery should be delayed as far as possible, preferably until the 4th week, when the necrotic process has stopped, and necrosis becomes localized and gets demarcated from viable tissue or walled-off necrosis (WON) forms. Necrosectomy at this stage is more likely to be complete and is associated with less risk of bleeding and injury to the adjacent bowel (colon or jejunum). Results of delayed (after 4 weeks) surgical intervention are much better (less mortality) than those of early surgical intervention.

DEPENDENT

An attempt must be made to make the internal drainage of a **pseudocyst** dependent as far as possible. For cysts in the lesser sac protruding into the posterior wall of the stomach, a **cystogastrostomy** will achieve this. For cysts below and inferior to the stomach and near the tail of the pancreas, cystogastrostomy may not be dependent and **cystojejunostomy** is preferable. Cysts near the head of the pancreas may be better drained into the duodenum—**cystoduodenostomy**.

DEROOFING

Areas of necrosis in the retroperitoneum need to be deroofed for complete **necrosectomy**; this may require mobilization of the right (ascending) and left (descending) colon.

DETERMINANT

Pancreatitis Across Nations Clinical Research and Education Alliance (PANCREA) including pancreatologists (including the author) from 49 countries proposed a new determinant-based classification of severity of acute pancreatitis in 2012. The determinants used are necrosis, infection (of necrosis), and organ failure. This classification includes four grades of severity of acute pancreatitis:

1. Mild (no necrosis AND no organ failure)
2. Moderate (sterile necrosis AND/OR transient organ failure)
3. Severe (infected necrosis OR persistent organ failure)
4. Critical (infected necrosis AND persistent organ failure).
   (Dellinger EP et al. 2012)

DIAGNOSIS

Diagnosis of acute pancreatitis can be made if any two of three viz. clinical, biochemical, or imaging (US, CT, or MRI) features are present. Classical clinical picture (acute onset severe persistent epigastric pain radiating to the back with nausea and vomiting) and elevated (>3 times normal) serum **amylase/lipase** is characteristic of acute pancreatitis. CT scan is not required for diagnosis of acute pancreatitis in majority of cases, especially if both clinical features and biochemical findings are present; it may be required if only pain is present and serum amylase is normal. CT is required for assessing the severity of acute pancreatitis and to detect local complications. CT, however, should be obtained if a surgical cause of **acute abdomen** cannot be excluded.

DIC

Disseminated intravascular coagulation (DIC) can occur in severe acute pancreatitis as a part of multiple organ dysfunction syndrome (MODS). This is caused by trypsin which activates prothrombin to thrombin. Diagnosis of DIC is suggested by:

Platelets <100,000/dL Fibrinogen <1 g/L

Fibrin degradation products (FDP) >80 μg/mL

DIET

A polymeric diet is well tolerated by patients with acute pancreatitis as an oligomeric or elemental diet which is more expensive.

DIFFERENTIAL DIAGNOSIS

Acute pancreatitis is a great mimic. Pain of acute pancreatitis may mimic that of many other acute abdominal conditions. Some patients with coronary artery disease (angina and myocardial infarction) and basal pneumonia or pleurisy may have upper abdominal pain and may be misdiagnosed as acute pancreatitis. Acute pancreatitis should be considered as a differential diagnosis in all patients with **acute** (upper) **abdomen**. Acute pancreatitis is quite often misdiagnosed as **peptic ulcer perforation**, acute cholecystitis, intestinal obstruction, intestinal perforation and peritonitis, acute mesenteric ischemia (AMI), leaking/ruptured abdominal aortic aneurysm (AAA), and **aortic dissection** or vice versa.

When dealing with an **acute abdomen**, more important than arriving at an accurate diagnosis is to decide whether it is a "surgical" acute abdomen, e.g., perforation—peritonitis, intestinal obstruction, AMI, or a "medical" acute abdomen, e.g., acute pancreatitis, acute gastritis, acute cholecystitis.

DIGITAL

Digital exploration and removal of necrotic debris avoid the risk of **bleeding** during **necrosectomy**. **Finger** is the best "instrument" to differentiate between necrotic debris and viable tissue.

DISCONNECTED DUCT SYNDROME

In patients with external pancreatic fistula following acute pancreatitis, endoscopic treatment is likely to fail if the main duct is disrupted because of extensive necrosis of pancreatic head and neck so that the distal viable pancreas continues to secrete pancreatic juice; surgery (fistulo-jejunostomy or resection) may be required.

DISTAL PANCREATECTOMY

A **pseudocyst** in relation to the tail of the pancreas (Figure D.2) is best treated by distal pancreatectomy (spleen preserving, if technically possible).

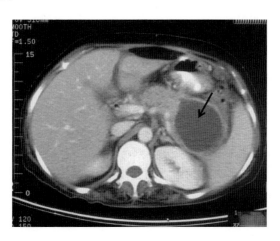

Figure D.2 Pseudocyst in tail of pancreas (amenable to excision by **distal pancreatectomy**).

DISTANT

Acute peripancreatic fluid collection (APFC) and acute necrotic collection (ANC) are usually peripancreatic but can be remote— distant from the pancreas, anywhere in the retroperitoneum.

DIVERTICULUM, PERIAMPULLARY

A periampullary diverticulum of the duodenum may cause recurrent acute pancreatitis by obstructing the pancreatic duct.

DIVISUM, PANCREAS

See **Pancreas divisum**

DOGMA

Several established dogmas, e.g., bowel rest, prophylactic antibiotics, early necrosectomy, etc., about acute pancreatitis are being challenged by new evidence.

D

DOPAMINE

An inotrope used in patients with hypotension due to MODS; in low doses (3–5 µg/kg/min), it improves the renal perfusion and function.

DOPPLER

Doppler US is a useful investigation for diagnosis of a **pseudoaneurysm** and splenic vein thrombosis (SVT)—both not uncommon vascular complications of acute pancreatitis.

DORIPENEM

Doripenem has more activity against pseudomonas than other **carbapenems**, e.g., **imipenem** and **meropenem**.

DRAINS

Drains placed percutaneously or surgically may erode into the vessels (causing bleeding) or the bowel (causing enterocutaneous fistula), especially if they are left in place for days/weeks. All drains must, therefore, be manipulated (rotated and/or shortened) at least once every few days.

DRUGS

A large number of drugs, e.g., steroids, azathioprine, nonsteroidal anti-inflammatory drugs (NSAIDs), diuretics (furosemide), valproic acid, ACE inhibitors, have been reported to cause acute pancreatitis.

DULL

The pain of acute pancreatitis is dull, continuous, and boring into the back, and lasts for hours (may be days).

DUODENAL ULCER

A posteriorly placed duodenal ulcer may penetrate into the pancreas and cause acute pancreatitis.

DUODENUM

D

A pseudocyst in close proximity to the second part of the duodenum (Figure D.3) is suitable for endoscopic drainage into the duodenum (endoscopic cystoduodenostomy).

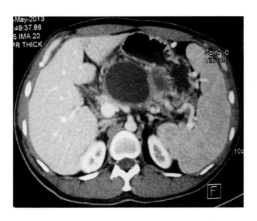

Figure D.3 A pseudocyst in close proximity to the second part of the duodenum.

DURATION

1. Prophylactic **antibiotics** given in patients with severe acute pancreatitis to prevent infection of necrosis should be given for 7–14 days.
2. Duration >6 weeks of an acute **pseudocyst** was earlier considered to be an indication for intervention. This is no longer true. Acute pseudocysts of duration >6 weeks can also be observed, if they are asymptomatic and do not have any complications. They can resolve on their own.

E

EARLY CT

Early (at admission) CT is indicated only if the diagnosis of acute pancreatitis is in doubt and surgical causes of **acute abdomen** cannot be ruled out. It may also be performed if a surgically correctable complication of acute pancreatitis, e.g., bleeding, gangrene, or perforation, is suspected.

EARLY GOAL-DIRECTED THERAPY

In patients with acute pancreatitis (as in those with sepsis and septic shock), early goal-directed therapy to maintain mean arterial pressure (MAP), central venous pressure (CVP), hematocrit (Hct), and ScvO$_2$ (central venous oxygen saturation) is of use.

EARLY ORGAN DYSFUNCTION

Early (cf. late) and persistent (cf. transient) organ dysfunction is a marker of poor prognosis in acute pancreatitis.

EARLY SURGICAL INTERVENTION

Early (within 2 weeks of onset of attack of acute pancreatitis) surgical intervention is hazardous—there is a higher risk of bleeding and bowel injury, necrosectomy is often incomplete and further intervention may be required, and mortality is much higher when compared with delayed (after 4 weeks of onset of attack of acute pancreatitis) surgical intervention. Early surgery may, however, be necessary for complications such as bleeding, ischemia, gangrene, and perforation.

ECG

ECG should be obtained in all patients with acute (upper) abdomen to rule out acute myocardial infarction (MI) which can present with upper abdominal (rather than chest) pain.

EDEMATOUS PANCREATITIS

A term used for **mild** acute pancreatitis—also called **interstitial** pancreatitis.

EEUS

US is a poor form of investigation for evaluation of the pancreas, especially in the presence of obesity and bowel gas. Echo-enhanced US (EEUS), after intravenous injection of SonoVue (an aqueous suspension of microbubbles), may be equal to or even better than CT in evaluating the pancreas. It is, however, not easily and universally available.

ELEMENTAL

Elemental enteral feeds containing monosaccharides, amino acids, and short-chain fatty acids (SCFAs) are preferred by some groups, but **polymeric** feeds are less expensive and as good.

EMBRYOLOGY

Pancreas develops as a dorsal and a ventral bud of the foregut. The ventral bud rotates and fuses with the dorsal bud to form the gland, with the dorsal bud forming the superior part of the head, body, and tail, and the ventral bud forming the inferior part of the head and the uncinate process. Failure of this rotation causes **annular pancreas** and failure of fusion causes **pancreas divisum**.

EMPHYSEMATOUS PANCREATITIS

Presence of gas (air) in and around the pancreas (without bowel perforation) indicates infected necrosis.

ENCAPSULATION

Encapsulation (localization) of acute peripancreatic fluid collection (APFC) to form pancreatic pseudocyst (PPC) and of acute necrotic collection (ANC) to form walled-off necrosis (WON) occurs at 4 weeks.

ENCEPHALOPATHY

Patients with severe acute pancreatitis may have disorientation, drowsiness, and altered sensorium, and may even be comatosed—this is due to the toxins released in acute pancreatitis.

E

ENDO GIA

Endo GIA^R stapler Covidien (45 mm, green, thick cartridge) can be used to perform laparoscopic **cystogastrostomy**—it creates a side-to-side stoma between the posterior wall of the stomach and the anterior wall of the **pseudocyst**.

ENDOSCOPIC INTERVENTION

EPT and biliary stenting (Figure E.1) may be useful if performed within 48–72 hours of onset of attack (*not* hospitalization) in a patient with severe (biliary) acute pancreatitis. It may also be performed in the presence of impacted stone with biliary obstruction

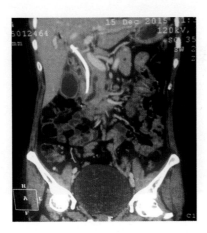

Figure E.1 **Endoscopic biliary stent** in situ.

and cholangitis. This should, however, be performed by an expert and experienced therapeutic endoscopist.

Pseudocyst and WON can also be managed endoscopically. Endoscopic drainage of pseudocyst can be transmural (transgastric or transduodenal) or transpapillary. WON can be removed using the transgastric route.

Late endoscopic intervention is indicated in patients with pancreatic ductal disruption, resulting in pancreatic leak (fistula and ascites).

ENDOSCOPIC MANAGEMENT

A pseudocyst in close approximation with the posterior wall of the stomach (Figure E.2) or the medial wall of the duodenum can be decompressed endoscopically (endoscopic **cystogastrostomy** or **cystoduodenostomy**).

The incision, made with a needle-knife papillotome, is dilated with a controlled radial expansion (CRE) balloon, and multiple pigtail stents or a nasocystic drain is placed into the pseudocyst. Endoscopic ultrasonography (EUS) is very helpful in avoiding

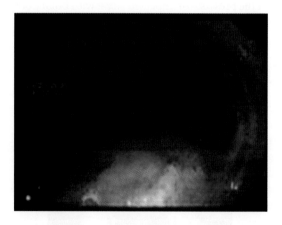

Figure E.2 Pseudocyst projecting into the stomach—suitable for **endoscopic management**.

the vessels and in puncturing the cyst at the most appropriate place. Endoscopic management is suitable for pseudocysts containing fluid only—those with necrotic debris (Figure E.3) are not suitable for endoscopic management and are better drained surgically. Endoscopic transpapillary drainage can be performed for a pseudocyst communicating with the main pancreatic duct.

E

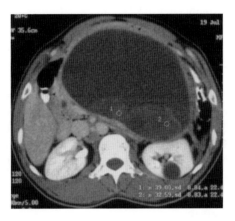

Figure E.3 Pseudocyst with some necrotic debris (1, 2)— not suitable for **endoscopic management**.

ENDOSCOPIC PAPILLOTOMY

1. Early (within 48–72 hours of the onset of the attack of acute pancreatitis) EPT may be helpful in patients with severe (biliary) acute pancreatitis with a common bile duct (CBD) stone impacted at papilla (indicated by high serum bilirubin or detected on MRC or EUS, if possible) with dilated CBD and biliary sepsis (cholangitis). This should, however, be done only by an experienced specialist.
2. Patients with acute biliary pancreatitis, who cannot undergo cholecystectomy for some reasons, should have an EPT to reduce the risk of recurrent attacks of acute pancreatitis.

ENDOSCOPIC TRANSGASTRIC NECROSECTOMY (ETN)

WON in the lesser sac can be removed endoscopically through the posterior wall of the stomach after dilating the opening with a CRE balloon. EUS can be very helpful to guide the procedure. A nasocystic drain is usually left for continuous lavage. Multiple sessions are usually required.

ETN for WON using balloon dilatation; bleeding and perforation of cavity are complications. EUS guidance helps in reducing the complications of the procedure.

ENDOSCOPIC TRANSPAPILLARY DRAINAGE

A pseudocyst communicating with the main pancreatic duct can be drained by passing an endoscopic nasopancreatic drainage tube through the papilla via the pancreatic duct into the pseudocyst after an EPT.

ENDOTOXINS

Increased permeability of the adjacent intestinal (colonic) wall due to inflammation results in translocation of endotoxins from the intestinal lumen to the peritoneal cavity where they are absorbed and cause MODS.

ENTERAL

A patient with mild acute pancreatitis should be kept nil by mouth (although sips of water can be allowed) for 2–4 days and can then be given oral fluids and feeds gradually; parenteral nutrition is not required. Enteral feeds can also be given to patients with severe acute pancreatitis through a nasogastric/nasojejunal tube unless the patient has severe paralytic ileus, active gastrointestinal bleeding, or suspicion of a bowel perforation (presence of air in the necrosis). Enteral feeds should be started after proper hydration and resuscitation—usually after 48–96 hours of admission.

Enteral (oral, nasogastric, nasojejunal, and feeding jejunostomy) nutrition is preferable to parenteral nutrition. Small enteral feeds can be given even in the presence of paralytic ileus. Patients with abdominal compartment syndrome (ACS) may not tolerate full enteral diet. Enteral feeds (even in small amounts) maintain the integrity of the gut mucosal barrier and reduce **translocation** of gut bacteria and **infection** of peripancreatic fluid collection/ necrosis. Some patients with acute pancreatitis may not tolerate oral feeds because of gastroparesis due to perigastric (especially retrogastric) inflammation. They may not tolerate nasogastric or nasoduodenal feeds also because of duodenal/jejunal inflammation and edema. A nasojejunal tube will be required to be placed to administer enteral nutrition in such cases.

E

ENTERIC FISTULA

An enteric fistula may be caused in acute pancreatitis as a result of necrosis of the bowel (colon, jejunum, or duodenum) wall caused either by the leaking pancreatic fluid or as a result of gangrene due to thrombosis of the mesenteric vessels. Damage may also occur to the bowel or to the vessels during surgery (necrosectomy) or can be caused by the drains.

Colon (transverse, right, and left) or proximal jejunum may form part of the wall of the necrosis/**abscess** and may give way easily either spontaneously or following intervention. Patients with proximal jejunal fistula are difficult to manage as it is usually a high-output proximal fistula. A **feeding jejunostomy** may be performed distal to the fistula and the fistula effluents may also be refed along with enteral feeds. In patients with colonic fistula, a proximal **ileostomy** must be performed as transverse colostomy is technically difficult/not possible because of inflamed thickened mesocolon and colonic wall. In case the colon is gangrenous with large areas of necrosis, colectomy (Figure E.4) may have to be performed.

Exposed bowel loops, as a result of **laparostomy**, may get traumatized during dressings and cause enteric fistula (Figure E.5). Such loops should be well covered with a nonadherent dressing.

E

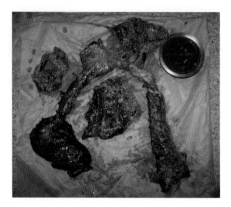

Figure E.4 Necrosectomy with subtotal colectomy and segmental resection of proximal jejunum.

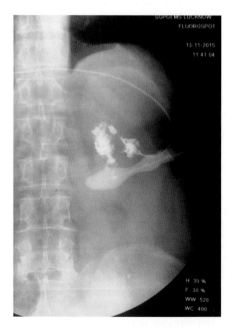

Figure E.5 Post-necrosectomy enteric fistula; fistulogram shows communication with distal transverse colon.

An enterocutaneous fistula may be treated conservatively if there is no peritonitis; a collection/abscess may be drained percutaneously. Fistula, especially colonic, is associated with high mortality—even higher, if associated **bleed** is also present.

ENTERIC ORGANISMS

Enteric organisms, i.e., Gram-negative bacilli (*Escherichia coli, Klebsiella*) and cocci (*Enterococcus*), are most frequently involved in **infection** of peripancreatic fluid collections/necrosis.

E

ENZYMES

1. Activation of pancreatic enzymes within the gland itself is an important event in the pathophysiology of acute pancreatitis. Inflamed pancreas releases several activated enzymes, e.g., amylase, lipase, elastase, trypsin, into the adjacent and surrounding tissues.
2. Serum levels of pancreatic enzymes, i.e., amylase and lipase, are elevated (>3 times normal) in the early phase of acute pancreatitis, but the levels of these enzymes have no correlation with the severity of acute pancreatitis.

EPF

See **External pancreatic fistula**

EPI

Extrapancreatic infections, e.g., pneumonia, urinary tract infection (UTI), lines.

EPIC (EXTRAPANCREATIC INFLAMMATION ON CT)

Extrapancreatic inflammatory changes, e.g., retroperitoneal and mesenteric inflammation, ascites, and **pleural effusion**, appear earlier than pancreatic changes (necrosis) on CT and may predict **severity** of the attack and development of **local complications** and **organ dysfunction**.

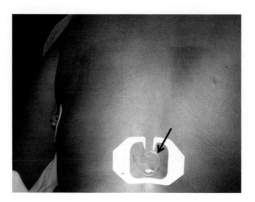

Figure E.6 **Epidural** catheter for analgesia.

EPIDURAL

Analgesia (patient controlled) through an epidural catheter (Figure E.6) is very effective in patients with acute pancreatitis.

EPITHELIAL LINING

Presence of epithelial lining in a true cyst differentiates it from a **pseudocyst** which has a wall of inflammatory granulation tissue and fibrous tissue and has no epithelial lining.

EPT

See **Endoscopic papillotomy**

ERCP (ENDOSCOPIC RETROGRADE CHOLANGIOPANCREATICOGRAPHY)

ERCP is indicated in patients with acute biliary pancreatitis only if the patient has CBD stones (Figure E.7) with obstruction, i.e., jaundice/cholangitis—papillotomy, stone extraction, and biliary stenting may be performed. Dilated CBD on US and rising liver enzymes may also indicate endoscopic biliary intervention in a patient with acute pancreatitis.

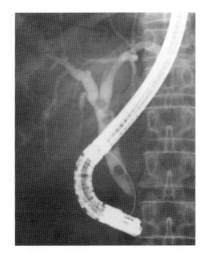

Figure E.7 ERC showing CBD stones.

ERCP-INDUCED ACUTE PANCREATITIS

Endoscopic retrograde cholangio-pancreaticography (ERCP) is not indicated in mild acute pancreatitis. ERCP is not indicated in severe acute pancreatitis without cholangitis also. ERCP can cause iatrogenic acute pancreatitis (post-ERCP acute pancreatitis)—more so when it is combined with an intervention, e.g., papillotomy (especially with a needle knife), stone removal, stenting, balloon dilatation of the sphincter, or pancreatic sphincterotomy.

Need for a pre-cut sphincterotomy, multiple attempts at canulation, pancreatic duct injection, and incomplete CBD clearance also increase the risk of acute pancreatitis.

Epigastric pain (new or worse), nausea, vomiting and elevated (>3 times normal) serum **amylase**, and **lipase** after ERC suggest acute pancreatitis. ERCP-induced pancreatitis can be severe (in about 10% of cases) and may even be fatal. Post-ERC, acute pancreatitis may be prevented by pre-ERC use of **octreotide** or **gabexate**, use of minimal amount of contrast, and placement of 5 Fr stent in the pancreatic duct, in high-risk cases.

ESBL

Many Gram-negative bacteria produce extended spectrum beta lactamase (ESBL) enzymes which hydrolyze and inactivate beta lactam **antibiotics** (including cephalosporins)—**carbapenems** have to be used in such cases.

ETHICAL ISSUES

Management of patients with severe acute pancreatitis poses several complex ethical issues because of its benign nature and, therefore, chances of the patient becoming normal on complete recovery but unpredictable (almost malignant) clinical course of the disease and high costs and mortality of treatment.

ETIOLOGY

Acute pancreatitis has a very diverse etiology. Two common causes of acute pancreatitis are **gallstone disease** (including **microlithiasis**) and **alcohol**. The next large group is **idiopathic** (no cause can be found). Less common causes include **trauma, tumors, metabolic disorders**, e.g., **hypertriglyceridemia and hypocalcaemia, drugs, viral infections**, and **pancreas divisum**.

Etiological workup includes detailed history (alcohol, drugs, trauma, family history), US (for gallstones), lab tests (lipid profile, serum calcium, etc.), EUS (for microlithiasis, chronic pancreatitis, small tumor), and MRCP (for chronic pancreatitis, pancreas divisum).

Endoscopic interventions, e.g., ERCP and EPT, can cause iatrogenic acute pancreatitis.

ETIOPATHOGENESIS

Zymogen granules that contain inactivated enzymes and lysosomes that contain hydrolases come together and result in intraacinar activation of pancreatic enzymes. The resulting parenchymal inflammation results in rupture of ductules, thus releasing the pancreatic enzymes into the peripancreatic tissues.

EUS

1. EUS plays an important role in the determination of etiology of **idiopathic / recurrent** acute pancreatitis by diagnosing small stones in the lower (retroduodenal/retropancreatic) CBD or biliary **sludge/microlithiasis**. EUS is more sensitive than MRC in detecting CBD stones but is semi-invasive and requires special equipment and expertise. It may also reveal a small pancreatic (periampullary) cancer, show early changes of chronic pancreatitis, and diagnose **pancreas divisum**.
2. EUS guides the location of the cyst, its distance from the stomach/duodenum, wall thickness (maturity), contents (fluid or solid necrotic debris), and shows the presence of collaterals and pseudoaneurysm when **endoscopic drainage** of a pseudo-cyst is being performed.

EXACERBATION

Preexisting comorbidities, e.g., diabetes, coronary artery disease (CAD), congestive heart failure (CHF), chronic obstructive pulmonary disease (COPD), chronic liver disease (CLD), may get exacerbated during an attack of acute pancreatitis.

EXAMINATION

Abdominal examination may reveal distension, tenderness, rigidity, and diminished bowel sounds in a patient with acute pancreatitis—all features of any **acute abdomen**.

EXTENT

An immediate preoperative, contract-enhanced CT scan delineates the extent of necrosis and serves as a road map to achieve complete necrosectomy.

E

Extensive necrosis (>50% of the gland) is predictive of organ dysfunction. Infection of extensive necrosis is associated with as high as 70% mortality.

EXTERNAL DRAINAGE

Fluid collections, **pseudocysts** with immature thin fragile walls, and infected pseudocysts (earlier called **abscesses**) cannot be drained internally and need external drainage. This should be performed by percutaneous radiological intervention, whenever possible. This, however, may result in an external pancreatic fistula (EPF).

EXTERNAL PANCREATIC FISTULA

An EPF (Figure E.8) is defined as >50–100 mL amylase-rich (>10,000 U/ mL) discharge persisting for more than 5 days (after an intervention—percutaneous or surgical). An internal pancreatic fistula causes pancreatic ascites and pleural effusion.

Drainage (percutaneous/surgical) of peripancreatic fluid collections results in a (transient) EPF; fistulae following acute pancreatitis will invariably close spontaneously since there is no distal obstruction (cf. chronic pancreatitis); they may, however, take months to close—*in one of our patients, the EPF following*

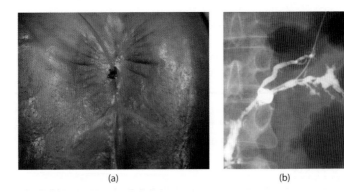

(a)   (b)

Figure E.8 External pancreatic fistula (EPF) after necrosectomy; (a) infant feeding in the fistulous opening in skin and (b) fistulogram showing communication with the main pancreatic duct.

necrosectomy *closed after 18 months.* Somatostatin analogue (**octreotide**) combined with TPN may hasten the closure of a pancreatic fistula. A persistent EPF following acute pancreatitis needs evaluation of the pancreatic duct—this can be done by a fistulogram, MRP, or ERP. Endoscopic intervention—pancreatic sphincterotomy and placement of a stent in the pancreatic duct across the site of disruption hastens the closure of the EPF. Rarely, a surgical fistulo-jejunostomy or resection of distal pancreas may be required for a persistent EPF.

EXTRAPANCREATIC

Lesser sac, transverse mesocolon, peri and pararenal spaces, mesentery of the small bowel, and retroperitoneum are some of the extrapancreatic areas involved in acute pancreatitis.

F

FAMILIAL

Mutation in trypsinogen gene predisposes even its carriers to acute pancreatitis.

FASCIA

See **Gerota's fascia**

FATAL

Age >70 years, **BMI** >30, **Ranson** score >5, **APACHE** II score >10, CT **necrosis** > 50%, **Balthazar** score >7, and infected necrosis are predictors of high mortality in acute pancreatitis.

FAT NECROSIS

Small (1–2 mm) whitish-yellow nodules on the omentum, peritoneum, mesentery, and serosa suggest a diagnosis of acute pancreatitis if a patient with suspected acute surgical abdomen is explored.

FEEDING JEJUNOSTOMY

Feeding jejunostomy (FJ) is preferred by some surgeons over a **nasojejunal** tube. FJ should be performed at the last abdominal exploration to avoid accidental detachment during one of the reexplorations. It is important to remember that the jejunal loop may be inflamed and edematous, and sutures may easily cut through.

FEVER

Fever in pancreatic necrosis does not necessarily mean infection of the necrosis as it may be fever due to inflammation caused by systemic inflammatory response syndrome (SIRS). Patients with acute pancreatitis may have fever because of urinary, chest, and catheter-related infections also. In patients with acute pancreatitis of biliary etiology, fever may be because of acute cholecystitis or acute cholangitis.

F

FFP

Fresh frozen plasma (FFP) to correct the coagulopathy of multiple organ dysfunction syndrome (MODS).

FINGER

For open surgical necrosectomy, fingers are the best instruments; suction tip, sponge holder, and Duval's forceps can also be used to remove necrotic debris.

FiO$_2$

Fraction of inspired oxygen content—for basic oxygenation; FiO$_2$ is usually kept at 0.5.

FISTULA, COLONIC

See **Colonic fistula**

FISTULA, ENTERIC

See **Enteric fistula**

FISTULA, PANCREATIC

See **External pancreatic fistula**

FITZ

Reginald Huber Fitz (Boston Medical and Surgical Journal, 1889) described 53 patients with acute pancreatitis and classified acute pancreatitis into hemorrhagic, gangrenous, and suppurative, based on autopsy findings.

FLUCONAZOLE

Patients with severe acute pancreatitis are immunocompromised and are prone to **fungal** infections. Some groups use prophylactic **fluconazole** to prevent these fungal infections.

FLUID COLLECTION

Collection of **amylase**-rich fluid in the peripancreatic areas with no defined wall peripancreatic fluid collection is an early (<4 weeks) event in the course of acute pancreatitis—it indicates severe acute pancreatitis. These fluid collections, which may be multiple (Figure F.1), are usually present adjacent to the pancreas but may be present in remote (Figure F.2) areas also. They do not have a well-defined wall (cf. **pseudocyst**, which has a wall of inflammatory granulation tissue and fibrosis).

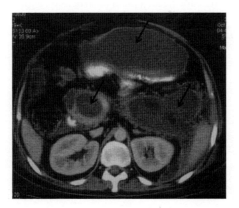

Figure F.1 Multiple **fluid collections** in acute pancreatitis.

F

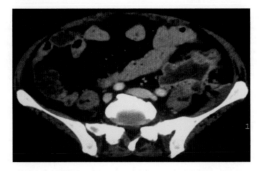

Figure F.2 Remote (lower abdomen) **fluid collection** in acute pancreatitis.

Most peripancreatic fluid collections do not require any intervention as they resolve spontaneously. A peripancreatic fluid collection is sterile to begin with but may get infected by **translocation** of bacteria through the inflamed gut wall to become what was earlier called an **abscess**; such an abscess usually contains pus only (and no necrotic debris) and is eminently suitable for percutaneous catheter drainage (PCD). A sterile fluid collection may also require drainage if it is causing pain or pressure symptoms, e.g., early satiety, postprandial fullness, and nausea due to a lesser sac fluid collection; gastric outlet obstruction/biliary obstruction due to a fluid collection around the pancreatic head, jejunal obstruction (Figure F.3).

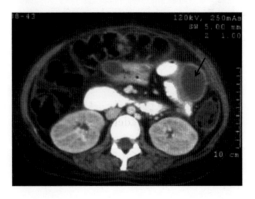

Figure F.3 **Fluid collection** (arrow) causing jejunal obstruction.

A ruptured fluid collection may result in pancreatic **ascites**.

Most fluid collections following acute pancreatitis resolve sponta-neously; some (10%–30%) may persist beyond 4–6 weeks and acquire a wall of granulation/fibrous tissue and mature into a **pseudocyst**.

FLUID REQUIREMENT

Patients with acute pancreatitis may require up to 3–5 liters of fluids (crystalloids and colloids) per day to maintain an adequate urine output; close watch, however, has to be kept in patients with cardiac, pulmonary, and renal dysfunction. Fluid administration should be monitored with central venous pressure (CVP), urine output, and hematocrit (Hct).

High (>4–5 liters/day) fluid requirement to maintain hemo-dynamic stability in the first few days of acute pancreatitis is a marker of poor outcome.

Early appropriate fluid resuscitation decreases the risk of per-sistent SIRS and organ failure in acute pancreatitis.

FLUOROQUINOLONES

See **Quinolones**

FNA

Fine-needle aspiration or FNA (under US or CT guidance) and gram staining of the smear is the only definite way to establish the presence of infection in pancreatic necrosis. FNA should be performed at least 7–14 days after the onset of the attack.

Most groups, however, do not perform FNA as a routine and guide their intervention based on other markers of infection, viz., fever, C-reactive protein, procalcitonin, imaging (presence of air/gas in necrosis), and clinical deterioration.

FOLLOW-UP

Some groups perform routine (weekly) follow-up CTs in patients being managed for severe acute necrotizing pancreatitis for early detection of local complications, especially pseudoaneurysm.

Patients with severe acute pancreatitis, especially those who have undergone necrosectomy, should remain under long-term follow-up to detect development of pseudocyst and external pancreatic fistula (EPF), obstruction of the common bile duct (CBD) and/or pancreatic duct due to fibrosis, and endocrine (diabetes) and exocrine (steatorrhea) deficiency.

FULMINANT

Patients with acute pancreatitis who start with a severe attack with early MODS have a fulminant course and poor outcome.

FUNGAL

Long-duration use of broad spectrum antibiotics and central venous catheters may predispose patients with acute pancreatitis to fungal sepsis which requires treatment with systemic **antifungal** agents.

There is no evidence to support routine use of **antifungal** prophylaxis with azoles, e.g., **fluconazole** or ketoconazole in patients with severe acute pancreatitis; many groups, however, use them to prevent fungal sepsis in patients with severe acute pancreatitis.

G

GABEXATE

Gabexate mesilate—an inhibitor of **protease**—has NOT been found to be of use in acute pancreatitis. It may, however, help to reduce the incidence of acute pancreatitis induced by endoscopic retrograde cholangiography (ERC).

GALLSTONES

Gallstone disease is the commonest cause of acute pancreatitis. Patients with multiple small stones in the gall bladder and a wide cystic duct are more likely to have common bile duct (CBD) stones and develop acute pancreatitis.

GANGRENOUS PANCREATITIS

A term used in the earlier classification of acute pancreatitis—not used now.

GAS

Presence of gas (**air**) in the necrotic tissue on CT is an evidence of **infection** of **necrosis** with gas-forming bacteria or bowel **perforation**—both indications for **intervention**.

GASTRIC OUTLET OBSTRUCTION

Inflammatory edema in the head of the pancreas may cause gastric outlet obstruction manifesting as retching, nausea, and vomiting.

GASTROCOLIC OMENTUM

The gastrocolic omentum has to be opened completely to expose the lesser sac adequately for a complete **necrosectomy**.

It is important to keep in mind that tissues are inflamed, edematous, and vascular, and it is not uncommon and unusual to cause inadvertent iatrogenic injury to the stomach, duodenum, or the transverse colon. It is always safer to remain close to the stomach than to the transverse colon.

GASTROINTESTINAL BLEEDING

See **Bleeding, Gastrointestinal**

GAUZE

A gauze piece mounted on a sponge holder (Figure G.1) can be used to remove necrotic debris during open necrosectomy.

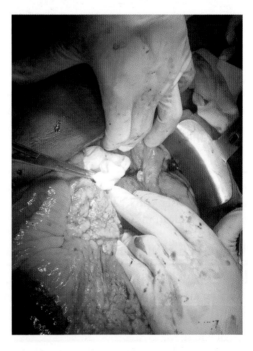

Figure G.1 Gauze piece mounted on sponge holder being used during necrosectomy.

GENES

Mutation of trypsinogen, serine protease inhibitor kajal (SPINK), and **cystic fibrosis** transmembrane regulator (CFTR) gene may be associated with acute pancreatitis.

GEROTA'S FASCIA

Inflammation in acute pancreatitis may involve the anterior para-renal (left more common than right) space and is seen as perirenal fat stranding and edematous thickening of the anterior perinephric (Gerota's) fascia (Figure G.2).

G

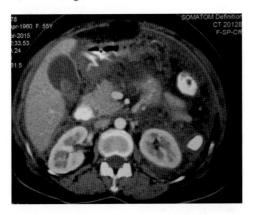

Figure G.2 Perirenal (left) fat stranding and thickened **Gerota's fascia** on the left side in acute pancreatitis; fat stranding is seen in the lesser sac; note the large gallstone also.

GI BLEEDING

See **Bleeding, Gastrointestinal**

GLASGOW (IMRIE) SCORE (1987)

C.W. Imrie of Glasgow, UK, proposed a modification of the **Ranson** criteria as follows: During the first 48 hours—WBC >15,000, blood glucose >10 mmol/L, blood urea >16 mmol/L, pO$_2$

<60 mm Hg, serum calcium <2.0 mmol/L, LDH >600 µ/L, ALT/AST >200, and serum albumin <3.2 g/L

GLUCOSE

Glucose is an important component of **parenteral nutrition**; it should contribute about 50%–70% of total calories.

GLUTAMINE

When **parenteral nutrition** is being given to patients with severe acute pancreatitis, glutamine supplementation should be considered.

GLYCEMIC CONTROL

Patients with severe acute pancreatitis (especially those with a background of chronic pancreatitis) may have **hyperglycemia** and require frequent monitoring of blood glucose and tight glycemic control (blood glucose between 4.4 and 6.1 mmol/L) with **insulin**.

GOAL DIRECTED

Targets of fluid therapy can be:

- Clinical—heart rate <120/min, MAP 65–85 mm Hg, urine output 0.5–1.0 mL/Kg/hour
- Biochemical—Hct 35%–45%

  This usually comes to 5–10 mL/Kg/hour

GOLD STANDARD

Contrast-enhanced CT scan is the gold standard investigation for diagnosis, assessment of the severity, and detection of necrosis in acute pancreatitis.

GPE (GENERAL PHYSICAL EXAMINATION)

Patients with acute pancreatitis, especially severe acute pancreatitis, look sick and have altered sensorium, fever, tachycardia, hypotension, and tachypnea (rapid and shallow breathing).

GRAM STAIN

In the presence of pancreatic/peripancreatic necrosis, Gram staining (Figure G.3) of the material obtained by image (US or CT)-guided fine-needle aspiration (FNA) is a useful test to diagnose infection. This is usually done in the 2nd or 3rd week of acute pancreatitis. Presence of infection is an indication for intervention.

G

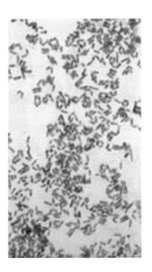

Figure G.3 **Gram-stained** smear of FNA showing bacteria.

GREY TURNER SIGN

Bluish discoloration of the flanks in severe acute pancreatitis—*rarely seen in clinical practice.*

GROOVE PANCREATITIS

Inflammation confined to the duodeno-pancreatic groove (Figure G.4), mainly in the upper part of the head of the pancreas. It may present as recurrent acute pancreatitis. On CT, it is difficult to differentiate from pancreatic head cancer. Pancreatic resection, which would be performed in most of the cases due to suspicion of pancreatic cancer, is difficult.

G

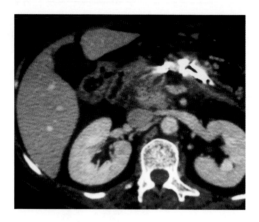

Figure G.4 Groove pancreatitis—inflammatory edema in the triangle between the duodenum, pancreas, and CBD.

GUIDELINES

Several scientific societies have, from time to time, formulated guidelines for the management of acute pancreatitis. There are more than 30 such guidelines; some of the important ones are (*Most of these are available for free on PubMed*):

- American College of Gastroenterology (ACG) Practice Guidelines. Tenner. *Am J Gastroenterol 2013; 108: 1400–1415.*
- American Gastroenterology Association (AGA) Institute Medical Position Statement. *Gastroenterology 2007; 132: 2019–21.*

- British Society of Gastroenterology (BSG) UK Guidelines. *Johnson. Gut 2005; 54 Suppl 3; 1–9.*
- International Association of Pancreatology (IAP)/American pancreatic Association (APA). Pancreatology 2013; 13: e1–e15—**the best guideline, in the Author's opinion**
- Japanese Society of HPB Surgery. *Hirota. J HBP Surg 2015; 22: 405–432.*

Guidelines are, however, not fully followed in real-life clinical practice: e.g., fine-needle aspiration (FNA) is recommended but not used; prophylactic antibiotics are not recommended but used.

G

H

HDU

Patients with severe acute pancreatitis should be managed in a high dependency unit (HDU) with facilities for noninvasive monitoring (pulse, blood pressure BP, central venous pressure or CVP, SpO$_2$, ABG analysis, etc.). Patients with respiratory dysfunction who may require ventilatory support may need to be shifted to an intensive care unit (ICU).

HEMATOCRIT

Hematocrit (Hct) >45%, which fails to fall even after fluid resuscitation within 24 hours, predicts the presence of **necrosis**/multiple organ dysfunction syndrome (MODS) in a patient with acute pancreatitis. Hct should be measured at admission and after 12 and 24 hours in all cases.

HEMOCONCENTRATION

Hemoconcentration caused by fluid loss in the retroperitoneum, manifested as raised hematocrit (Hct), is a strong indicator of the presence of necrosis in acute pancreatitis.

HEMODYNAMIC INSTABILITY

Patients with severe acute pancreatitis may develop hemodynamic instability (hypotension and shock) as a part of MODS. Adequate fluid resuscitation with inotropic support, if required, is a key factor in the early management of acute pancreatitis.

HEMORRHAGE

Sudden severe pain with increase in the size of a preexisting **pseudocyst** indicates hemorrhage into the pseudocyst as a result of erosion of an adjacent vessel, e.g., splenic, middle colic or gastroduodenal artery, or rupture of a **pseudoaneurysm** into the cyst. Angiographic **embolization** of the pseudoaneurysm is the treatment of choice. If it fails, surgical intervention is required—it involves ligation of the vessel which, however, may be difficult in the presence of inflammation.

HEMORRHAGIC PANCREATITIS

A term used in the earlier classification of acute pancreatitis—not used now.

HEMOSUCCUS PANCREATITIS

Rupture of a **pseudoaneurysm** into the pancreatic duct presenting as pain, jaundice, melena, and blood coming out of the duodenal papilla as seen on side-viewing endoscopy (SVE). Angiographic **embolization** of the pseudoaneurysm is the treatment of choice. If it fails, surgical intervention is required—it involves ligation of the vessel which, however, may be difficult in the presence of inflammation.

HEREDITARY

Hereditary acute pancreatitis is defined as acute pancreatitis in childhood and two family members affected. Mutation of trypsinogen gene is often present.

HES

Hydroxyethyl starch (HES) is discouraged for resuscitation as it increases the risk of renal dysfunction.

HIV

Patients with HIV infection and AIDS are more prone to develop acute pancreatitis.

HOSPITAL STAY

Patients with mild acute pancreatitis can be discharged from the hospital in few (3–7) days. Those with severe, especially necrotizing, acute pancreatitis need to stay in the hospital for weeks, may be even months.

HYDRATION

Patients with acute pancreatitis are usually dehydrated (high hematocrit, or Hct) due to poor intake and loss of volume in the third space. They should be well hydrated with crystalloids before CT is done to reduce the renal toxicity of the IV contrast used during CT.

H

HYPERCALCAEMIA

Hypercalcaemia may be a cause of **recurrent** acute pancreatitis. Patients with recurrent acute pancreatitis should be investigated to detect hypercalcaemia and its cause, e.g., hyperparathyroidism.

HYPERCATABOLIC

Patients with severe acute pancreatitis are in severe **catabolism** and have very high calorie and protein requirements.

HYPERGLYCEMIA

Patients with severe acute pancreatitis may develop hyperglycemia due to transient insulin deficiency because of endocrine dysfunction. Blood glucose levels should be closely monitored.

HYPERLIPIDEMIA

Hyperlipidemia may be a cause of **recurrent** acute pancreatitis. Patients with recurrent acute pancreatitis should have a complete lipid profile to detect hyperlipidemia.

HYPERPYREXIA

Patients with acute pancreatitis can develop malignant hyperpyrexia which can even cause death.

HYPERTENSION, DUCTAL

Pancreatic ductal hypertension caused by obstruction plays an important role in the pathogenesis of acute pancreatitis.

HYPERTENSION, INTRAABDOMINAL

See **Intraabdominal hypertension**

HYPERTRIGLYCERIDEMIA (HTG)

Triglyceride level >1000 mg/dL suggests hypertriglyceridemia to be the cause of acute pancreatitis. Xanthomas are characteristic. Serum may appear grossly milky (lactescent). Treatment includes dietary fat restriction, weight reduction, and lipid-lowering drugs.

HYPOCALCAEMIA

Patients with severe acute pancreatitis may develop hypocalcaemia due to consumption of calcium in the process of saponification of fat. Serum calcium levels should be monitored and corrected, if low.

HYPOPERFUSION

Hypoperfusion of the gland should be avoided/corrected in a patient with acute pancreatitis to prevent progression to necrosis. Hypoperfusion can occur due to hypotension.

HYPOTENSION

1. Severe and persistent hypotension of any cause can cause pancreatic hypoperfusion and acute pancreatitis.

2. Some patients with acute pancreatitis, especially severe acute pancreatitis, may have peripheral vasodilatation and high cardiac output (as seen in patients with septic shock)—restoration of volume in such cases may not correct hypotension, and vasoconstrictors may be required.

HYPOMAGNESAEMIA

Hypomagnesaemia can occur in patients with severe acute pancreatitis. It can be corrected by administration of magnesium sulfate.

H

HYPOTHERMIA

Hypothermia can cause acute pancreatitis due to hypoperfusion of the gland.

HYPOVOLEMIA

Third space fluid loss can cause severe hypovolemia in the early phase (1st week) of acute pancreatitis. This should be corrected by guided administration of fluids and colloids.

HYPOXIA

Hypovolemia and hypoxia should be avoided/corrected in a patient with acute pancreatitis to prevent progression to necrosis.

HYPOXEMIA

Patients with acute pancreatitis may have hypoxemia due to **atelectasis**. SpO_2 should be monitored and oxygen should be administered (using mask or nasal prongs).

I

IAH (INTRAABDOMINAL HYPERTENSION)

Intraabdominal pressure is measured with a urinary bladder catheter—IAH can cause abdominal compartment syndrome (ACS). IAH is defined as intraabdominal pressure >15 mm Hg. If the intraabdominal pressure becomes >25 mm Hg, it is defined as ACS.

IATROGENIC

Acute pancreatitis can be an iatrogenic disease following endoscopic retrograde cholangiography (ERC), especially if the pancreatic duct is repeatedly canulated and after endoscopic papillotomy (EPT), biliary manometry, and cardiopulmonary bypass.

ICU

Society of Critical Care Medicine (CCM) for admission of a patient to ICU/HDU recommends the following criteria (any one or more):

- Pulse <40/min or >150/min, systolic arterial pressure (SAP) <80 mm Hg, mean arterial pressure (MAP) <60 mm Hg, respiratory rate >35/min
- Serum Na <110 mmol/L or >170 mmol/L, serum K <2.0 mmol/L or >7.0 mmol/L, serum Ca >15 mg/mL
- pH <7.1 or >7.7, PaO_2 <50 mm Hg
- Serum glucose >800 mg/dL
- Anuria (urine output <100 mL in 24 hours)

IDIOPATHIC

In a significant proportion (about 20%) of cases of acute pancreatitis, no etiological cause can be found even after extensive investigations—this is idiopathic acute pancreatitis. Many patients labeled as "idiopathic" acute pancreatitis may, however, be biliary, as small stones, **microliths** and **sludge** may have passed out of the papilla. Duodenal bile aspiration and analysis for crystals may help in such cases.

IDIOPATHIC RECURRENT ACUTE PANCREATITIS

Endoscopic ultrasonography (EUS) has become the investigation of choice (in place of ERCP) for idiopathic recurrent acute pancreatitis.

ILEOSTOMY

Colon (usually transverse) often forms part of the wall of the necrotic cavity. If at the time of necrosectomy, the colon looks precarious (giving way) or if there is lot of pericolitis, a diverting proximal loop ileostomy (Figure I.1) should be performed.

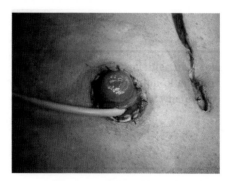

Figure I.1 **Ileostomy** may be required when the transverse colon is involved in acute pancreatitis; note the Foley's catheter placed in the distal ileal loop for refeeding

ILEUS

Patients with severe acute pancreatitis may develop paralytic ileus as a part of multiple organ dysfunction syndrome (MODS).

Majority of patients with severe acute pancreatitis have paralytic ileus—**enteral feeds**, however, should not be withheld on this ground alone. Even patients with paralytic ileus may tolerate enteral (nasogastric or nasojejunal) feeds, albeit i ı small amounts.

IMAGE INTENSIFIER

Image intensifier is required for minimally invasive retroperitoneal necrosectomy (MIRN)/video-assisted retroperitoneal debridement (VARD).

IMIPENEM

Imipenem, a **carbapenem** (combined with cilastin) (500 mg–1 g every 6 hours) is an antibiotic of choice for use in patients with severe acute pancreatitis.

IMMUNONUTRITION

Immunonutrition is an attractive option for patients with severe acute pancreatitis but more evidence needs to be generated to recommend its routine use.

IMPENDING ORGAN FAILURE

Patients with impending organ failure should receive **organ support** in a high dependency unit (HDU) or intensive care unit (ICU) to prevent full blown multiple organ failure (MOF).

IMRIE

See **Glasgow (Imrie) score (1987)**

INCIDENCE

Incidence of acute pancreatitis is about 10–20 per 100,000 population per year in USA and Europe, and it seems to be increasing. Acute pancreatitis is responsible for about 200,000 admissions in

USA costing about US$ 2.5 billion every year. Acute pancreatitis is the most common gastroenterological discharge diagnosis in the USA.

INCISION

Choice of incision for necrosectomy depends on the body habitus of the patient and the extent of necrosis as seen on CT. An upper midline incision can be used for necrosectomy in some patients. Bilateral subcostal bucket handle incision may be better in short and stout patients with a wide costal angle. Patients with extensive infracolic, mesenteric, and retroperitoneal necrosis should be explored with a long midline incision.

INCISIONAL HERNIA

An incisional hernia very commonly forms during long-term follow-up in patients who underwent a laparotomy for necrosectomy because wound complications, viz., infection and dehiscence are frequent.

INDEX

In a patient with acute biliary pancreatitis, cholecystectomy can (should) be performed in the index admission only, before the patient is discharged from the hospital. Interval cholecystectomy (after 4–6 weeks) is not preferred as it is associated with a risk of a recurrent attack of acute pancreatitis while waiting.

INDICATIONS FOR INTERVENTION

Persisting/deteriorating organ functional status in spite of intensive **organ support** is an indication for intervention.

Demonstration of infection of necrosis (positive fine-needle aspiration FNA or presence of **air** in necrosis) is an indication for intervention (though there are several anecdotal reports of successful conservative management of even infected pancreatic necrosis).

INDICATIONS FOR SURGERY

1. Uncertain diagnosis of an **acute abdomen** used to be an indication for surgery—with the easy and universal availability of CT and laparoscopy, this should be a rare situation today. If abdomen is opened with a diagnosis of acute surgical abdomen and acute pancreatitis is found, abdomen should be closed (without drains).
2. Early surgery may also be indicated for management of locoregional complications, e.g., **bleed**, bowel necrosis/gangrene, and **perforation**.
3. Infected necrosis
4. Persisting or worsening organ failure despite aggressive **organ support** (even if the necrosis is sterile)
5. Symptomatic walled-off necrosis (WON)
6. Abdominal compartment syndrome (ACS)

INFARCTION

Inflammatory thrombosis of splenic, jejunal, or middle colic artery may lead to infarction/gangrene of the spleen, jejunal, or colonic segment.

INFECTED NECROSIS

See **Infected pancreatic necrosis**

INFECTED PANCREATIC NECROSIS (IPN)

Pancreatic and peripancreatic necrosis, to begin with, is sterile. It gets infected due to **translocation** of gut (colonic) bacteria across the inflamed gut wall. One-third of patients with necrosis will get infected. Any intervention, percutaneous, endoscopic, or surgical, also causes infection of the necrosis. Infection of the necrosis increases the risk of morbidity and mortality of necrotizing pancreatitis. Mortality of infected necrosis is as high as 30% (cf. 10% in sterile necrosis). Chances of infection of necrosis increase with increasing duration of illness: 20%–30% in the 1st week, 30%–40% in the 2nd week, and 50%–60% by the 3rd week. Risk of infection is also proportional to the degree of necrosis: <30% necrosis—20% risk of infection, 30%–50% necrosis—40% risk of infection, and >50% necrosis—50% risk of infection. Infection of necrosis is the most important risk factor for mortality in severe acute pancreatitis.

Infection in pancreatic necrosis is diagnosed by US- or CT-guided fine-needle aspiration (FNA) and examination of the **Gram**-stained smear. FNA is highly specific but false-negative rates may be up to 20%–25%. SIRS, MODS, fever, and WBC count are markers of inflammation also and are not definite proofs of infection. C-reactive protein and procalcitonin have been used as surrogate markers of infection of necrosis.

Most patients with infected pancreatic necrosis (IPN) require some intervention but conservative management (with antibiotics) can be tried under close monitoring in stable patients.

INFECTED PSEUDOCYST

A pseudocyst with presence of infection in its contents was earlier classified as an **abscess**.

INFECTION

1. Several **viral** infections, e.g., mumps, measles, varicella, coxsackie B, infectious mononucleosis, HIV, can cause acute pancreatitis.
2. Definite diagnosis of infection of necrosis can be made on FNA only; fever and leucocytosis beyond 2 weeks are highly suggestive of infection.
3. Infection of pancreatic necrosis is the most important determinant of mortality in acute pancreatitis; mortality of infected necrosis being 30%–40% cf. 10% of sterile necrosis.

INFLAMMATION

In acute pancreatitis, inflammation is not synonymous with infection.

INITIAL

Initial management of acute pancreatitis involves fluids, oxygen, and analgesia.

INOTROPES

Inotropes (e.g., dopamine and dobutamine) should be administered in a patient with hypotension only after fluid deficit has been replaced and central venous pressure (CVP) has been restored.

INSECTICIDES

Organophosphorus insecticides can cause acute pancreatitis.

INSULIN

Patients with acute pancreatitis, especially those receiving parenteral nutrition where glucose is an important component, may develop **hyperglycemia** and need treatment with insulin (subcutaneous or preferably intravenous infusion).

INTENSIVISTS

All intensivists, even if they are from nonmedical nonsurgical background, should be familiar with the management of severe acute pancreatitis as most patients with severe acute pancreatitis need to be managed in HDU/ICU.

INTERNAL DRAINAGE

A **pseudocyst** has to be mature (thick walled) for internal drainage—this usually happens after 4–6 weeks. Internal drainage can be in the form of **cystogastrostomy, cystojejunostomy**, or **cystoduodenostomy**.

INTERSTITIAL

Mild acute interstitial pancreatitis (also called acute edematous pancreatitis).

INTERVAL

In patients with severe acute biliary pancreatitis, cholecystectomy should be performed after an interval of 4–6 weeks after all collections have resolved/stabilized and the patient is free of sepsis.

INTERVENTION

Intervention is almost never required in mild acute pancreatitis.

Intervention in acute pancreatitis can be endoscopic, percutaneous, radiological, or surgical.

Common indications for intervention in acute necrotizing pancreatitis are:

1. **Infection** of **necrosis**
2. Clinical deterioration
3. Persistent WON or WON causing biliary, gastro/duodenal, or intestinal obstruction

Rarely, early intervention may be required for ACS, **bleeding**, bowel ischemia, gangrene, and **perforation**.

INTESTINAL NECROSIS

Adjacent bowel (e.g., transverse colon or proximal jejunum) may undergo necrosis—this results in infection of peripancreatic necrosis or gastrointestinal **bleeding**. Prognosis in such cases is worse.

INTESTINAL OBSTRUCTION

Pain, vomiting, and distension of mechanical intestinal obstruction can mimic acute pancreatitis.

Colicky pain associated with and relieved by projectile vomiting, obstipation (inability to pass both feces and flatus), and abdominal distension with visible loops and peristalsis and exaggerated bowel sounds is characteristic of mechanical intestinal obstruction.

Abdominal X-rays show dilated bowel loops (supine) and multiple air fluid levels (erect).

Complete acute intestinal obstruction invariably needs surgical intervention.

INTRAABDOMINAL ABSCESS (IAA)

A residual IAA is a frequent complication after surgery for pancreatic necrosis. Patients who continue to have features of sepsis (e.g., fever, tachycardia, leucocytosis, unsettled abdomen, persisting/worsening organ dysfunction) should be suspected to have an IAA. US may be done as a screening bedside investigation but CT must almost always be obtained. Most of these abscesses can be managed with image (US or CT)-guided percutaneous catheter drainage (PCD); laparotomy is rarely required.

INTRAABDOMINAL HYPERTENSION

See **IAH**

IPN

See **Infected pancreatic necrosis**

IPPV

Intermittent positive pressure ventilation (IPPV)—the commonest mode of artificial respiration.

ISOAMYLASE, PANCREATIC

Differentiates it from salivary amylase.

J

JAUNDICE

Patients with acute pancreatitis may have jaundice due to:

1. Choledocholithiasis with or without cholangitis in patients with biliary acute pancreatitis
2. Inflamed edematous pancreatic head pressing on the lower end of the common bile duct (CBD)
3. Peripancreatic **fluid collection/pseudocyst** causing CBD obstruction
4. Alcoholic hepatitis in patients with alcoholic acute pancreatitis

JEJUNOSTOMY

See **Feeding jejunostomy**

JVP

Jugular venous pressure (JVP) in the neck veins may be used as a crude indicator of hydration status, especially raised JVP in overhydration—central venous pressure (CVP), however, is a better indicator.

L

LACTATE DEHYDROGENASE

Serum lactate dehydrogenase (LDH) >5 U/L indicates severe (necrotizing) acute pancreatitis.

LAPAROSCOPIC

1. In patients with acute pancreatitis of biliary etiology (laparoscopic), cholecystectomy will prevent recurrent attacks of acute pancreatitis. This may be done in the same hospital admission in patients with mild acute pancreatitis and after a few (4–6) weeks of resolution in patients with severe acute pancreatitis.
2. In patients with gallstones and CBD stones, laparoscopic CBD exploration may be done if expertise is available.
3. Internal drainage of **pseudocyst** and **necrosectomy** can be performed laparoscopically in selected patients with severe acute pancreatitis.

LAPAROSCOPIC CYSTOGASTROSTOMY

1. Transgastric approach after making an anterior gastrotomy. The opening into the cyst through the posterior wall of the stomach can be made with Harmonic scalpel and anastomosis can be done with suture; alternatively, a stapled anastomosis can be done between the posterior wall of the stomach and the anterior wall of the cyst using Endo GIA (Covidien/Medtronic) or Echelon (Ethicon).
2. Intragastric approach in which two working canulae are inserted into the stomach which has been inflated via an upper gastrointestinal endoscope (UGIE) placed in the stomach.
3. A posterior (lesser sac) approach is also used.

LAPAROSCOPIC US

Laparoscopic US, if available, is a useful tool to evaluate the common bile duct (CBD) for any stones during laparoscopic cholecystectomy in patients with acute (biliary) pancreatitis.

LAPAROSTOMY

Some surgeons/groups leave the abdomen open (laparostomy) after **necrosectomy** for easy planned reexploration. This, however, exposes the bowel loops and increases the chances of **fistula** formation. Planned reexplorations are more often required when necrosectomy is done in the early phase (1st–3rd week) of acute pancreatitis, when the necrotic process is not well localized and demarcation between necrotic and viable tissues is not clear. Complete necrosectomy is, therefore, not feasible and a reexploration (to remove residual/further necrosis) is "planned." The trend now is toward late necrosectomy (after 3rd or 4th week) when the necrotic process has well localized and demarcation between necrotic and viable tissues is clear. Complete necrosectomy is, therefore, possible and reexploration is not "planned"; reexploration is instead done on an SOS basis.

Laparostomy may be preferred if necrosectomy has to be done early, if it is thought to be incomplete, and if abdominal compartment syndrome (ACS) is present.

LATE

Surgical intervention in acute pancreatitis, whenever indicated, should be performed as late as possible (preferably in the 3rd or 4th week) so that the necrotic process is localized.

LAVAGE

Most surgeons/groups believe in **necrosectomy** to be followed by closed drainage with multiple (2–4) large-bore (28–36 F) silicone rubber drains (Figure L.1) and high-volume (6–12 liters/day) continuous lavage (Figure L.2) with normal saline to remove residual

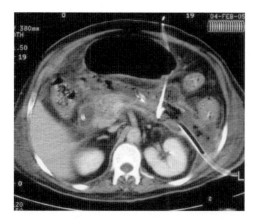

Figure L.1 Large-bore drains placed after necrosectomy for **lavage**.

L

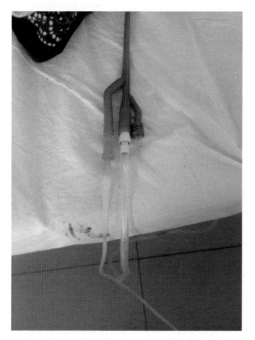

Figure L.2 Three-way Foley's catheter for lavage.

necrotic debris, infected fluid, and toxic substances. The opened lesser sac should be reclosed to isolate the supracolic lesser sac from the rest of the peritoneal cavity. Hyperosmolar potassium-free peritoneal dialysis fluid can also be used for lavage. Lavage is continued till the returns contain necrotic debris.

LDH

Serum LDH (lactate dehydrogenase) >5 U/L indicates severe (necrotizing) acute pancreatitis.

LEAK

Disruption of pancreatic duct in acute pancreatitis may cause leak of pancreatic juice, resulting in peripancreatic **fluid collection**, pancreatic **ascites**, and pancreatic **pleural effusion**.

LESS INVASIVE

Less (than conventional open surgical) invasive interventions for necrosis include extra (retro)peritoneal, laparoscopic, endoscopic, and percutaneous radiological interventions.

LESSER SAC

Lesser sac has to be opened by dividing the gastrocolic omentum for exposing the pancreas. In patients with severe peripancreatic inflammation, the lesser sac may be obliterated and the gastro-colic omentum may get thickened and shortened and may be very inflamed and vascular, thus making access to the lesser sac difficult and bloody; care must be exercised to avoid injury to the stomach, transverse colon, and the spleen. It is safer to remain close to the stomach than to the colon.

Lesser sac may also be approached through the inferior aspect of transverse mesocolon to the left of the middle colic artery.

Majority of pseudocysts form in the lesser sac and are, therefore, located behind the stomach and are amenable to internal drainage by **cystogastrostomy**.

LEXIPAFANT

Lexipafant, a platelet-activating factor (PAF) antagonist, has NOT been found to be of use in acute pancreatitis.

LFT (LIVER FUNCTION TESTS)

Deranged LFT (serum bilirubin, ALT/AST, and alkaline phosphatase) in a patient with acute pancreatitis suggest biliary etiology, although it must be remembered that inflammation and edema in the head of pancreas in acute pancreatitis of any etiology can cause compression of the CBD and result in deranged LFT. CBD obstruction can be caused by a pseudocyst in the head of the pancreas also.

LIFE THREATENING

Severe acute pancreatitis is a life-threatening disease. Although benign, it has a mortality higher than most cancers.

LIPASE

Serum lipase rises soon after (within 4–8 hours) the onset of acute pancreatitis—it peaks within 24 hours and remains elevated for 7–14 days (cf. serum **amylase** which settles within 3–5 days) and then returns to normal.

Elevated serum lipase is more specific for the diagnosis of acute pancreatitis than elevated serum **amylase**.

Elevation of both serum lipase and **amylase** in a patient with **acute abdomen** is almost diagnostic of acute pancreatitis.

Serum lipase level 2–3 times that of **amylase** suggests alcoholic pancreatitis.

LIPIDS

Lipids (0.8 to 1.5 g/Kg) are an important component of **parenteral nutrition** because of their high caloric value. Serum triglycerides, however, should be closely monitored and kept below 12 mmol/L.

LIQUEFACTION

With increasing time, necrosis liquefies, but walled-off necrosis (WON) contains significant amount of solid necrotic **debris**.

LIVER FUNCTION TESTS

See **LFT**

LONG-TERM COMPLICATIONS

Necrosis/removal of large volumes of necrotic pancreatic parenchyma during necrosectomy may result in endocrine (diabetes)/exocrine (steatorrhea) pancreatic insufficiency in the long term.

LUMP

An ill-defined tender abdominal lump (earlier called **phlegmon**) may be palpable in the upper abdomen in patients with acute pancreatitis. Pseudocyst may be palpable as a well-defined nontender lump.

M

MAGNITUDE

The incidence of acute pancreatitis in USA is 17 new cases per 100,000 per year; acute pancreatitis results in about 125,000 hospital admissions every year.

MAGNESIUM

Patients with acute pancreatitis may develop **hypomagnesaemia** and require administration of magnesium sulfate.

MALNUTRITION

Malnutrition may preexist at the time of admission in patients with acute pancreatitis, especially of alcoholic etiology. These patients may require **nutritional support** from the very beginning.

Obesity, on the other hand, is also associated with higher morbidity and mortality in acute pancreatitis.

MARKERS

C-reactive protein, interleukin 6, interleukin 8, tumor necrosis factor (TNF) alpha, and procalcitonin (PCT) are some of the markers of inflammation present in acute pancreatitis.

MARSEILLE CLASSIFICATION (1989)

Marseille classification of acute pancreatitis was pathological—edematous and necrotizing; it was replaced by **Atlanta** classification which is clinical and radiological.

Organ system	Score				
	0	1	2	3	4
Respiratory (PaO_2/FiO_2)	>400	301–400	201–300	101–200	<101
Cardiovascular (SAP, mm Hg)	>90	<90	<90	<90 pH <7.3	<90 pH <7.2
Renal (serum creatinine, umol/L)	<134	134–169	170–310	311–439	>439

MARSHALL SCORING SYSTEM

The revised Atlanta classification has used modified Marshall scoring system which includes three organ systems, viz., respiratory, cardiovascular, and renal. A score of 2 or more in any organ system defines organ failure.

MD CT

Multidetector (MD) CT gives better delineation of anatomy and allows 3-D reconstruction of the images. MDCT perfusion imaging provides excellent images of the pancreas.

MDF

Some patients with severe acute pancreatitis develop acute heart failure due to release of a myocardial depressant factor (MDF) from the inflamed pancreas.

MEDIATORS

Several mediators of inflammation (e.g., **cytokines**, bradykinins, endotoxins, nitric oxide, interleukins, and prostaglandins) are involved in the pathogenesis of acute pancreatitis.

MEDICAL

Acute pancreatitis in the first 2 weeks is a "medical" (nonsurgical) illness requiring intensive **organ support**.

MEROPENEM

Meropenem (1–2 G IV every 8 hours), a **carbapenem**, is the antibiotic of choice in patients with acute pancreatitis.

MESENTERIC INFLAMMATION

Release of pancreatic enzymes causes inflammation of the small bowel mesentery, seen as thickening, edema, and fat stranding (Figure M.1) on CT.

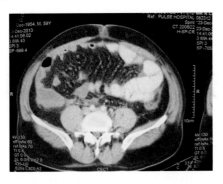

Figure M.1 Fat stranding in small bowel mesentery in acute pancreatitis.

MESOCOLIC APPROACH

If the lesser sac is obliterated and gastrocolic access is difficult, an inframesocolic approach may be used to access the lesser sac for necrosectomy.

METABOLIC DERANGEMENTS

Hyperglycemia, **hypocalcaemia**, and **hypomagnesaemia** can occur in patients with severe acute pancreatitis.

METABOLIC DISORDERS

Metabolic disorders, e.g., **hypercalcaemia**, **hyperlipidemia**, and **hypertriglyceridemia**, can cause acute pancreatitis.

M

MICROLITHS

Microliths, defined as small (<2–3 mm) stones not seen on US, are a frequent cause of acute pancreatitis.

Duodenal bile drainage and analysis (microscopy) should be performed in patients with **recurrent** acute pancreatitis in whom no gallstones (GS) are seen on US in order to detect microlithiasis or crystals as a cause of recurrent acute pancreatitis. Endoscopic ultrasonography (EUS) may be more sensitive than abdominal US to detect microliths in the lower common bile duct (CBD). Patients with microlithiasis can be managed with oral bile acids (lifelong), endoscopic papillotomy, or cholecystectomy.

MICROPERFORATION

Microperforations of the transverse colon are common in acute pancreatitis—they result in **infection** of peripancreatic **fluid collections** and **necrosis**.

MIDDLE COLIC VESSELS

Middle colic vessels often traverse the necrosis in the lesser sac and may get thrombosed because of inflammation, resulting in colonic gangrene and perforation. These vessels may also get damaged during **necrosectomy**, resulting in profuse intraoperative bleeding.

MILD

Majority (75%–80%) of patients with acute pancreatitis has a mild, self-limiting disease—they have an uneventful recovery with no/very little (<1%) mortality. Pathology of mild acute pancreatitis involves interstitial edema—there is no necrosis. It is also called **interstitial** or **edematous** pancreatitis. CT, if done, shows complete enhancement of the pancreas which may be edematous (Figure M.2); there are no local complications. Mild acute pancreatitis is acute pancreatitis with no organ dysfunction.

Treatment of mild acute pancreatitis includes hospitalization, nil by mouth, intravenous fluids, and **analgesics** (no antibiotics are required). Most attacks resolve within 5–7 days.

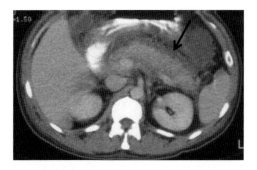

Figure M.2 Edematous gland in **mild** acute pancreatitis.

MIN

Minimally invasive necrosectomy.
    See also **MIPN**.

MINOR DUODENAL PAPILLA

M

Minor (accessory) papilla, located about 2 cm proximal to the major (main) papilla, drains the minor (accessory) pancreatic duct of **Santorini** (Figure M.3). It assumes importance in **pancreas divisum**.

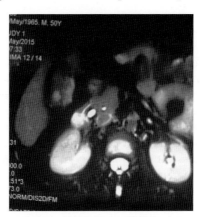

Figure M.3 Minor pancreatic duct opening into the duodenum above the major pancreatic duct.

MIPN

Minimally invasive pancreatic necrosectomy (MIPN) can be:

1. Laparoscopic—preferable for single fluid collection, advantage of simultaneous cholecystectomy
2. Retroperitoneal approach through a flank incision for left-sided fluid collection
3. Minimally invasive retroperitoneal necrosectomy (MIRN)—for necrosis around tail of pancreas
4. Endoscopic—for necrosis behind body of stomach

MIRN

Minimally invasive retroperitoneal necrosectomy—image-guided percutaneous catheter drainage (PCD) is performed, the tract is dilated, and a nephroscope is used for removing the necrotic material; multiple sessions are often required.

MIRPN

Minimally invasive retroperitoneal pancreatic necrosectomy—another name for MIRN.

MODERATE

Earlier, there was no entity called moderate acute pancreatitis; acute pancreatitis was classified as either **mild** or **severe**. Some groups suggested that the term "moderate acute pancreatitis" should be introduced as some patients with acute pancreatitis are more severe than mild acute pancreatitis and less severe than severe acute pancreatitis. The revised **Atlanta** classification introduced the category of moderate acute pancreatitis. These are patients with **local complications** but with no **transient organ failure** (no persistent organ failure); they have high morbidity but low (5%–10%) mortality.

MODS

Multiple organ dysfunction syndrome (MODS) is caused in the initial phase of acute pancreatitis as a result of release of toxins, vasoactive substances, and inflammatory mediators. In the later phase, it is caused as a result of sepsis due to infected necrosis.

MODS involves the dysfunction of more than one organ. Renal, pulmonary, and cardiac dysfunction have poorer prognosis as compared with dysfunction of other organs/systems, viz., gastrointestinal, coagulation, metabolic.

MONITORING

Frequent, regular, and intense (both clinical and laboratory) monitoring is the key to successful management of severe acute pancreatitis.

MORPHOLOGICAL

1. Morphologically, acute pancreatitis is classified into edematous (mild; 80%–90% of all cases) and necrotizing (severe; 10%–20% of all cases).
2. A morphological change can occur in the pancreatic duct after an attack of acute pancreatitis causing stricture and chronic pancreatitis (CP).

MORTALITY

Patients with mild acute pancreatitis should not have any mortality; on the contrary, severe acute pancreatitis is associated with high (up to 25%) mortality, especially in the presence of **necrosis, infection**, and MODS.

MRCP

It is a must to obtain a magnetic resonance cholangio-pancreaticogram (MRCP), and may be an endoscopic ultrasonography (EUS), in order to rule out biliary stone disease (including microlithiasis), chronic pancreatitis, and pancreas divisum before labeling a patient as idiopathic acute pancreatitis. MRCP is less sensitive than EUS in detecting CBD stones but is noninvasive, less operative dependent, and more easily available.

	Mortality (%)
Mild (edematous) pancreatitis	<1
Moderate pancreatitis	5–10
Severe (necrotizing) pancreatitis	10–40
Sterile necrosis	5–10
Infected necrosis	30–40

Note: Acute pancreatitis/necrosectomy is a disease/ procedure with one of the highest rates of mortality.

MRI

More and more centers are using magnetic resonance imaging
(MRI) in place of CT for evaluation of severe acute pancreatitis.
Gadolinium-enhanced, T1-weighted MRI can differentiate peripancreatic fluid from **necrosis** and blood. T2 images can show
fluid collection and **pseudocyst** (Figure M.4).

M

MRI is safer than CT in patients with renal dysfunction and
also provides an opportunity to obtain an MRCP to evaluate the

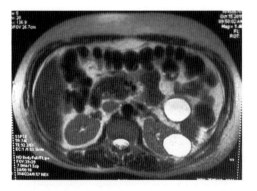

Figure M.4 MRI T2-weighted image showing a hyperintense
pseudocyst behind the stomach; the other hyperintense lesion
behind the pseudocyst is an incidental renal cyst.

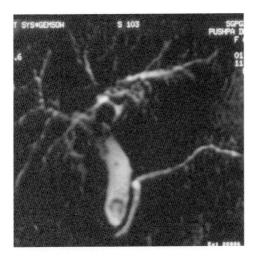

Figure M.5 MRCP showing CBD stone.

biliary tree for CBD **stones** (Figure M.5) and pancreatic duct (for **pancreas divisum** and underlying chronic pancreatitis).

M

MRI is better than CT to detect solid necrotic debris in a fluid collection. Presence of significant amount of solid necrotic debris differentiates acute necrotic collection (ANC) from acute peripancreatic fluid collection (APFC) and walled-off necrosis (WON) from pancreatic pseudocyst (PPC).

MULTIDISCIPLINARY

Patients with severe acute pancreatitis should preferably be managed by a team comprising gastroenterologist, surgeon, radiologist, and intensivist.

MULTIPLE

Both APFC and ANC can be single or multiple (Figure M.6); they can, however, be drained together (Figure M.7) if they are communicating with each other.

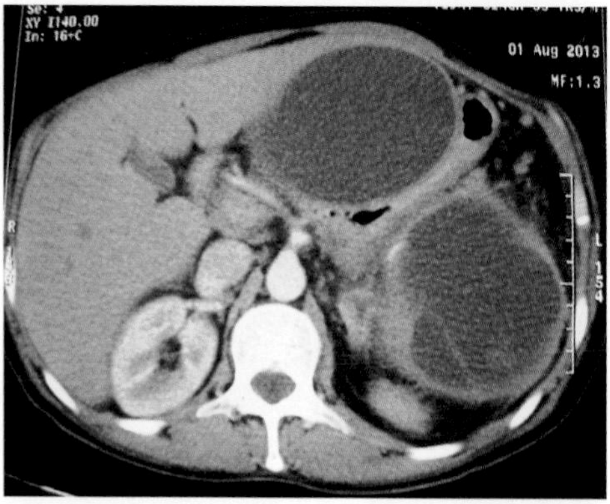

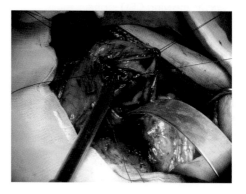

Figure M.6 Multiple (2) pseudocysts, one anterior and one posterior to the stomach (Courtesy of Prof. Anu Behari).

M

Figure M.7 Both cysts got drained with a single cystogastrostomy as they communicated with each other (Courtesy of Prof. Anu Behari).

N

NAC (N-ACETYL-L-CYSTEINE)

N-acetyl-L-cysteine (NAC) is used to protect the kidneys when using IV contrast for CT in patients with renal dysfunction. It is to be started the day before CT and should be continued for 48 hours after CT.

NASAL PRONGS

Oxygen may be administered with nasal prongs or a mask.

NASOCYSTIC

A nasocystic drain can be left into the pseudocyst after endoscopic drainage for continuing drainage, irrigation, and lavage.

NASOGASTRIC TUBE

Nasogastric tube may help patients with acute pancreatitis by taking care of nausea and vomiting. In addition, aspiration of gastric acid may decrease pancreatic enzyme secretion. In later stages, it may be sued for administration of **enteral** feeds.

NASOJEJUNAL

Some patients with lesser sac inflammation/fluid collection/necrosis may not tolerate oral or nasogastric feeds because of either mechanical gastric outlet obstruction (GOO) or inflammatory **gastroparesis**; a nasojejunal tube should then be placed under fluoroscopic guidance for **enteral feeding**.

NAUSEA

Patients with acute pancreatitis usually have nausea, vomiting, and retching along with **pain**. This is because of the retrogastric inflammation.

NECROSECTOMY

Necrosectomy is the removal of peripancreatic and pancreatic nonviable devitalized necrotic debris with preservation of normal viable pancreatic parenchyma (Figure N.1). It can be surgical (open laparotomy, open retroperitoneal, laparoscopic or video-assisted retroperitoneal debridement [VARD]), percutaneous radiological, or endoscopic.

It is important to keep in mind that the necrotic process may extend beyond the pancreas into the base of the small bowel mesentery, transverse mesocolon, and perinephric and retrocolic spaces. It is difficult to ascertain the extent of retroperitoneal necrosis at operation and, therefore, it is absolutely necessary to have a good contrast-enhanced CT just before the operation.

Necrosis is seen/felt as black or brown, thick, soft, putty-like or spongy material. Some pus may also be present along with the necrotic debris.

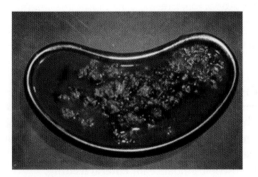

Figure N.1 Necrotic debris and pus removed during **necrosectomy**.

Necrosectomy is done as a blunt dissection with **finger**, sponge holder, and suction tip; sharp dissection with knife, scissors, or cautery is best avoided.

Following necrosectomy, the patient invariably ends with multiple tubes including drains for lavage and feeding jejunostomy (Figure N.2).

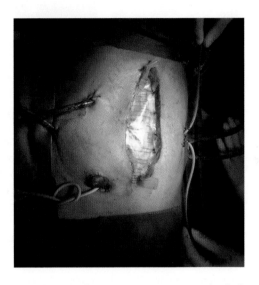

N

Figure N.2 Abdomen after necrosectomy—multiple large-bore portex drains (feeding jejunostomy, loop ileostomy with a Foley's in distal loop for refeeding, laparostomy with temporary closure of skin with a plastic patch.

NECROSIS

Focal or diffuse areas of nonviable pancreatic parenchyma—seen as nonenhanced or poorly enhanced (normal pancreas parenchyma has a density of 100–150 HU) areas on contrast-enhanced CT (Figure N.3). Necrosis can be pancreatic or peripancreatic. Peripancreatic necrosis can be retroperitoneal, mesenteric, transverse mesocolic, perirenal, paracolic, and retrocolic; it can

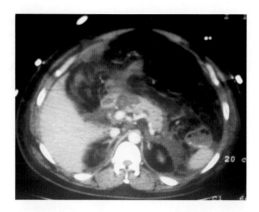

Figure N.3 Contrast-enhanced CT showing patchy area of **necrosis** in the neck of pancreas.

be focal or diffuse. Peripancreatic necrosis is difficult to detect on CT as normal fat also does not have much enhancement. Most patients have both pancreatic and peripancreatic necrosis, some have peripancreatic necrosis alone, and rarely only pancreatic necrosis is seen.

In addition to solid necrotic debris, some liquid pus may also be present as a result of liquefaction of the necrotic tissue (Figure N.4). Necrosis may not be seen on CT in the first 48–72 hours. Presence of necrosis on CT indicates severe acute pancreatitis. The **extent** of necrosis has a bearing on the occurrence of **organ failure** and the risk of **infection**.

Necrosis is the most important predictor of **mortality**. Patients with necrosis (on CT) have 20% mortality (cf. no mortality in patients with no necrosis). Half of these deaths occur early in the course of acute pancreatitis due to organ failure; the remaining half occurs later due to local complications. More than half of the patients with necrotizing acute pancreatitis have organ failure.

Adjacent bowel, e.g., colon or jejunum, may necrose because of the action of proteolytic and lipolytic pancreatic enzymes or as a result of vascular thrombosis.

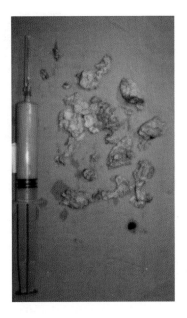

Figure N.4 More necrosis and little pus in pancreatic **necrosis**.

N

NEPHROSCOPE

Image-guided percutaneous extraperitoneal access is obtained to the necrotic cavity—the tract is dilated and an operating nephroscope is used for removal of the necrotic debris and irrigation of the necrotic cavity—minimally invasive retroperitoneal necrosectomy (MIRN).

NIPPV

Noninvasive positive pressure ventilation, e.g., CPAP.

NONCONTRAST

In patients with renal dysfunction, a noncontrast CT may be done though it does not provide much information; an MRI may be better.

NOSOCOMIAL

Patients with severe acute pancreatitis, especially those who require intervention, have prolonged hospital stay and are at risk to develop nosocomial (hospital acquired) infections.

NPI

Nonpancreatic infections (NPIs), e.g., pneumonia and urinary tract infection (UTI), are more common in the first 1–2 weeks (cf. infection of necrosis after 2–3 weeks).

NUTRITION

It is very important to look after nutrition in patients with acute pancreatitis. As far as possible, **enteral nutrition** is preferred over **parenteral**. Enteral feeding is less expensive, easier to administer, has less complications, and maintains the integrity of the gut mucosa, thus decreasing bacterial **translocation** and infection of fluid collection/necrosis.

NUTRITIONAL STATUS

Nutritional status of the patient should be assessed at the time of admission and then frequently (every 5–7 days) to determine the need of nutritional support.

NUTRITIONAL SUPPORT

Nutritional support would be required in patients with preexisting **malnutrition** or if oral intake is not possible or is inadequate for about 5–7 days. Patients with severe acute pancreatitis are similar to patients with systemic sepsis, extensive burns, and polytrauma in terms of their nutritional requirements. All patients with acute pancreatitis should receive daily dose of multivitamins and trace elements.

O

OBESITY

Obese patients (BMI >30) have a poorer prognosis (higher mortality) after an attack of severe acute pancreatitis. A modification of **APACHE II—APACHE O**—includes obesity as a risk factor.

OBSTRUCTION

Obstruction of the pancreatic duct/ampulla/ sphincter of **Oddi**, e.g., due to common bile duct (CBD) stone/**microliths/sludge**, causes acute biliary pancreatitis.

OCTREOTIDE

Octreotide, a somatostatin analogue, has no role in the management of acute pancreatitis. It may, however, prevent post-ERC acute pancreatitis. It may also be used along with total parenteral nutrition (TPN) in the management of pancreatic **ascites** and external pancreatic fistula (EPF). Dose is 100 μg SC q8h.

ODDI, SPHINCTER OF

The common channel formed by the union of the pancreatic duct and the CBD is surrounded by a sphincter (of Oddi) which, in some cases, may be long and extend beyond the duodenal wall. Endoscopically, only the intramural (intraduodenal) part of the sphincter can (should) be divided. That is why, the author prefers to call it endoscopic papillotomy (EPT) and NOT sphincterotomy; sphincterotomy can be performed surgically only in the form of transduodenal sphincteroplasty (TDS).

ON DEMAND LAPAROTOMY

Relaparotomy after **necrosectomy** only as and when indicated by either clinical course or based on CT findings (cf. **planned** relaparotomy).

ONSET

Organ dysfunction early in the course of acute pancreatitis indicates a worse prognosis and higher mortality. Surgery in the form of necrosectomy may not be helpful in such cases, especially if the necrosis is sterile.

OPEN

1. If laparoscopic necrosectomy is being planned, open technique of insertion of the first port should be used as bowel is usually distended due to paralytic ileus.
2. Open technique of insertion of the first port during laparoscopic cholecystectomy in a patient with acute (biliary) pancreatitis is safer because of the high likelihood of presence of adhesions of omentum and bowel loops to the anterior abdominal wall.

OPEN PACKING

Some surgeons prefer to leave the abdomen open (**laparostomy**) (Figure O.1) after **necrosectomy**—the necrotic cavity is packed

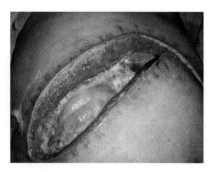

Figure O.1 Abdominal wound after **open packing** (laparostomy).

with a nonadherent sheet separating the pack from the walls of the cavity; this makes reoperation and repeat dressings easier. This can be done even on the bedside in the ICU on a patient on ventilator. Open packing is, however, associated with increased risk of bleeding and **fistula** formation; **incisional hernia** is inevitable.

ORAL FEEDS

Oral feeds can be resumed in patients with mild acute pancreatitis when pain and fever have subsided, nausea has improved, and bowel activity has returned, usually within a few days of the onset of the attack.

ORGAN FAILURE

Cardiovascular	Shock, systolic BP <90 mm Hg
Respiratory	PaO_2 <60 mm Hg
Renal	Serum creatinine >2 mg/dL (after rehydration)
Gastrointestinal	Bleeding >500 mL/24 h
Coagulation (DIC)	Platelets <100,000/dL
	Fibrinogen <1g/L
	Fibrin degradation products (FDP) >80 μg/mL

APACHE score (>8), Ranson score >3, modified Glasgow score >3, and SOFA score >4 are predictors of organ dysfunction.

Early and adequate correction of hypovolemia and hypoxemia may prevent or delay the onset of organ failure.

The time of onset of organ failure, viz., early (within 3 days) due to SIRS or late (after 7 days) due to sepsis, is important as early organ failure is associated with higher mortality.

Duration of organ failure, viz., transient (<48 hours) or persistent (>48 hours) is also important as patients with transient organ failure usually recover without other complications, whereas persistent organ failure is associated with higher mortality. Organ failure which occurs in the first week of illness and resolves within 48 hours after providing organ support (responsive) does not increase the mortality of acute pancreatitis. Failure of multiple organs is associated with higher mortality than single organ failure. Which organ is involved is also important, with mortality being higher in respiratory, renal, cardiovascular, coagulation, neurological, and GI failure, in that order.

ORGANIZED NECROSIS

Necrosis which over a period of time (usually 4–6 weeks) has become localized (now called walled-off necrosis, or WON) and separated from the normal viable tissue and is easy to remove surgically.

ORGANISMS

Both bacteria (aerobes and anaerobes) and fungi are involved in sepsis related to acute pancreatitis and should be looked for.

ORGAN PRESERVATION

The philosophy of surgical management of acute pancreatitis has changed from aggressive resection to conservative organ (pancreas) preservation.

ORGAN SUPPORT

Patients with severe acute pancreatitis require support for multiple organs/systems in an HDU/ICU.

OVUM FORCEPS

Ovum forceps is a useful blunt instrument to remove the necrotic tissue during **necrosectomy**.

OXYGEN

Oxygen should be administered by nasal prongs or face mask to patients with acute pancreatitis to prevent **hypoxia**.

Oxygen saturation should be monitored and maintained at >95%. Arterial blood gases (ABGs) should also be monitored in patients with severe acute pancreatitis.

P

PACKING

Packing (Figure P.1) may be required after **necrosectomy** if the residual cavity has continuous ooze from its walls. This is more likely to happen if an early (1–2 weeks) surgical intervention has been performed and the necrosis was not well demarcated. Pack should be removed after 24–48 hours; packs which remain in situ for >48 hours may get infected.

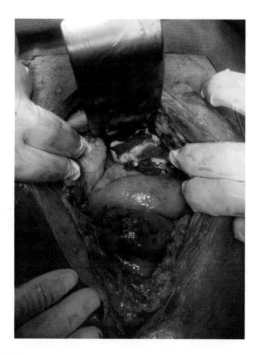

Figure P.1 Bleeding necrotic cavity being packed with roller gauze soaked in povidone and iodine.

PaCO$_2$

Arterial partial pressure of CO_2 (normal upper limit 40 mm Hg).

PAIN

Almost all patients with acute pancreatitis have pain. It is usually in the epigastrium/upper abdomen (left more than right) but may be generalized. It is insidious at onset (cf. peptic ulcer perforation where the onset of pain is sudden); dull, steady, continuous, deep, boring, severe (usually unbearable); and lasts for hours to days; it may radiate to the back (or chest or flank) and get relieved by sitting up or curling or bending forward. A large, heavy fatty meal or a binge of alcohol may precipitate an attack. Pain of acute pancreatitis is usually associated with nausea and vomiting.

Pain is the predominant symptom in patients with acute pancreatitis. All patients with acute pancreatitis should receive adequate pain relief with adequate **analgesia**.

It must, however, be noted that the severity of pain does not correlate with the severity of pancreatitis.

PANCREA

PANCREA (Pancreatitis across Nations Clinical Research and Education Alliance) of pancreatologists (including the author) from 49 countries proposed a new determinant-based classification of severity of acute pancreatitis in 2012. The **determinants** used are necrosis, infection (of necrosis), and organ failure. This classification includes four grades of severity of acute pancreatitis—mild (no necrosis AND no organ failure), moderate (sterile necrosis AND/OR transient organ failure), severe (infected necrosis OR persistent organ failure), and critical (infected necrosis AND persistent organ failure) (Dellinger EP et al. 2012).

PANCREAS DIVISUM

Pancreas develops as a ventral bud and a dorsal bud protruding from the foregut. Ventral bud of the pancreas originates from the ventral diverticulum which forms the liver, gall bladder, and the common bile duct. Dorsal bud of the pancreas arises directly from the duodenum. The ventral bud rotates around the duodenum to fuse with the dorsal bud to lie inferior to it. The ventral bud forms the inferior part of the head and the uncinate process of the pancreas. The dorsal bud forms the superior part of the head, neck, body, and tail of the pancreas. The lumen of the ventral bud forms the main pancreatic duct (of Wirsung) while that of the dorsal anlage forms the minor pancreatic duct (of Santorini).

Failure of the two ducts (dorsal duct of **Santorini** and ventral duct of **Wirsung**) to unite results in pancreas divisum. Major (ventral) duct of **Wirsung** then drains only the inferior part of the head and the uncinate process; most of the pancreas (superior part of the head, neck, body, and tail) is drained by the minor (dorsal) duct of **Santorini** through the minor papilla (Figure P.2)—which may be inadequate for drainage of major proportion of pancreatic juice, thus resulting in relative obstruction and causing **recurrent** acute pancreatitis. Pancreas divisum is present in 5%–10% of population but does not cause acute pancreatitis in everyone.

Patients with recurrent acute pancreatitis, in whom no obvious cause is found on routine investigations, should be investigated (magnetic resonance pancreaticography, or MRP; endoscopic retrograde pancreaticography, or ERP; and endoscopic ultrasonography, or EUS) for pancreas divisum which can cause recurrent acute pancreatitis.

Pancreas divisum can be treated by endoscopic papillotomy or surgical sphincteroplasty of the minor papilla.

P

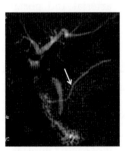

Figure P.2 **Pancreas divisum** on MRCP—body and tail of pancreas are drained by the "minor" pancreatic duct (arrow) which becomes more prominent.

PANCREAS PROTOCOL

Helical CT with thin (<5 mm) sections taken through the pancreas during bolus (3–5 mL/seconds) administration of about 100–150 mL of IV contrast (preferably nonionic) with a dual head injector; triple-phase scanning with arterial (20–25 seconds), parenchymal (35–45 seconds), and portal venous (50–60 seconds) phases. Pancreatic parenchyma is best seen at 50–60 seconds.

PANCREATIC ABSCESS

See **Abscess, Pancreatic**

PANCREATIC ASCITES

See **Ascites, Pancreatic**

PANCREATIC FISTULA

See **External Pancreatic Fistula**

P

PANCREATIC PHASE

Pancreatic phase on CT can be obtained by imaging about 45 seconds (between arterial and portal venous phases) after injection of IV contrast.

PaO$_2$

Arterial partial pressure of oxygen—normal 100 mm Hg.

PARACENTESIS

Paracentesis (aspiration of ascitic fluid) is not recommended for diagnosis of acute pancreatitis. It may, however, help in diagnosis of intraabdominal bleed and perforation—peritonitis. In the presence of ascites, however, examination of the peritoneal fluid (for amylase) is essential to make a diagnosis of **pancreatic ascites**.

PARATHYROID

While investigating the etiology of **recurrent** acute pancreatitis, if **hypercalcaemia** is found, parathyroid glands should be investigated as the cause of hypercalcaemia.

PARENTERAL NUTRITION

Patients who do not tolerate **enteral** feeds may have to be given parenteral nutrition.

Parenteral nutrition can be started once the patient has been resuscitated and is hemodynamically stable (usually 24–48 hours of admission).

Patients who are denied enteral nutrition for a long time develop atrophy of the intestinal mucosa, resulting in compromise of the gut barrier and **translocation** of gut (colonic) bacteria to the peritoneal cavity/retroperitoneal tissues.

PASS

Most patients with acute biliary pancreatitis will have stones in their common bile duct (CBD) at some point in time, but in the majority of the patients these stones will pass down through the papilla into the duodenum—for this reason, not all patients with acute biliary pancreatitis require endoscopic intervention on the CBD.

PATHOGENESIS

The pathogenesis of acute pancreatitis remains obscure. The final common pathway seems to be acinar rupture, resulting in activation of trypsinogen and chymotrypsinogen causing autodigestion of pancreatic tissue. This causes release of pancreatic **enzymes**, e.g., amylase, lipase, protease, elastase, into the surrounding tissues.

PATHOLOGY

Pathology of acute pancreatitis ranges from parenchymal edema, inflammation, and microscopic to gross necrosis.

PATHOPHYSIOLOGY

Basic pathophysiological process in acute pancreatitis is the activation of pancreatic **enzymes** causing autodigestion of the pancreatic parenchyma and the peripancreatic tissues.

PCA (PATIENT-CONTROLLED ANALGESIA)

Pain (often severe) is an important and usually the only symptom in patients with acute pancreatitis. Relief of pain is an important component of treatment of acute pancreatitis. PCA with narcotics is a good practice and is very useful in patients with acute pancreatitis. This can be intravenous or epidural (see PCEA).

PCD (PERCUTANEOUS CATHETER DRAINAGE)

Image (US or CT)–guided percutaneous catheter drainage (PCD) plays an important role in the management of complications of severe acute pancreatitis. A **fluid collection** may be aspirated (with a needle) or drained (by a catheter) if it is infected or is causing obstruction (gastric, jejunal, or biliary). An **abscess** may also be definitively drained percutaneously. In patients with **necrosis**, PCD of the infected fluid/pus may control the ongoing sepsis, improve **organ failure**, and buy some time so as to delay surgery (**necrosectomy**). PCD is very useful to drain residual/recurrent fluid collections after surgery.

Multiple drains (Figure P.3) may have to be placed for multiple or multiloculated fluid collections; large (24–28 F) drains may be required for solid necrotic debris; irrigations are liberally used. Dormia basket and snare catheter may be used to remove solid necrotic debris. Complete resolution after PCD may take 10–14 days, or even longer.

PCD may avoid the need of surgical **necrosectomy** in some cases. Failure of PCD is an indication for surgery.

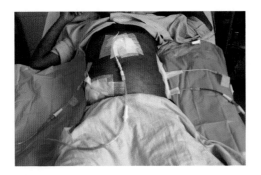

Figure P.3 Multiple PCDs.

PCEA

Patient-controlled epidural analgesia.
    See also **PCA**.

PCT

See **Procalcitonin**

PCWP

Pulmonary capillary wedge pressure (PCWP) is a better indicator of volume/hydration status than central venous pressure (CVP), especially in patients on ventilatory support.

PEAKS

Two peaks of death occur in acute pancreatitis—the first (early; 1–2 weeks) due to SIRS and MODS and the second (late; 3–4 weeks) due to **infection** of the necrosis and septic complications.

PEEP

Positive end-expiratory pressure ventilation—useful in the management of ARDS.

PENETRATION

Antibiotics with good penetration into the pancreatic tissue such as **carbapenems** and **fluoroquinolones** are preferred in patients with acute pancreatitis.

PEPTIC ULCER

A posteriorly placed peptic (duodenal) ulcer can penetrate into the pancreas and cause acute pancreatitis.

PERFORATED PEPTIC ULCER

Peptic ulcer perforation is one of the common causes of acute abdomen and can mimic acute pancreatitis. It is important to differentiate between the two because while acute pancreatitis needs medical management, perforated peptic ulcer needs urgent surgical intervention.

Duodenal ulcer perforation is more common than gastric ulcer perforation. The patient may give history of symptoms of peptic ulcer disease (PUD; acid dyspepsia) or NSAID intake, but not all patients with peptic ulcer perforation have previous symptoms of PUD.

Presentation is with severe and sudden (so sudden that the patient can tell the exact time when the pain started) onset pain in the epigastrium or the right hypochondrium; vomiting is not a predominant symptom. Guarding, rigidity, and tenderness are present and liver dullness may be obliterated on percussion.

Free air under the domes of the diaphragm (seen best on a chest X-ray in sitting or standing position) clinches the diagnosis. CT with oral (and IV) contrast may have to be obtained in some cases to settle the diagnosis.

Most patients with peptic ulcer perforation will need urgent surgical intervention for closure of the perforation; few (with localized perforation) may be managed conservatively.

PERIPHERAL

It is not essential to have a central venous catheter (CVC) to administer **parenteral nutrition**. Several parenteral nutrition preparations are available which are suitable for peripheral venous administration. Peripheral administration of parenteral nutrition is, however, associated with thrombophlebitis and the lines may have to be changed frequently.

PERITONITIS

1. With pain, vomiting, distension, guarding, and paralytic ileus, acute pancreatitis may mimic acute peritonitis.
2. An infected pseudocyst may rupture into the free peritoneal cavity and cause peritonitis (to be differentiated from **pancreatic ascites** caused by rupture of a sterile pseudocyst).

PERMEABILITY

Intestinal permeability is increased in patients with acute pancreatitis resulting in bacterial **translocation** from the gut (colon) to the peritoneal cavity resulting in **infection** of **necrosis**.

PERSISTING

Persistent, i.e., >48 hours (cf. transient, i.e., <48 hours) SIRS/**organ failure** is associated with very high (up to 50%) mortality in acute pancreatitis.

pH

Low pH (and **base deficit**) as seen on ABG is a marker for poor outcome in acute pancreatitis.

PHASES

Severe acute pancreatitis has two phases of the disease—early (1–2 weeks) toxic phase (SIRS and MODS caused by **cytokine** cascade) and late (after 3–4 weeks, extending for several weeks, sometimes even months) septic (**necrosis** and **infection**) phase. Treatment in early phase is largely conservative and supportive; intervention may be required in the late phase.

PHLEGMON

A term used in earlier classification to describe an inflammatory mass including the inflamed pancreas and peripancreatic organs/tissues— not used now. These patients have acute necrotic collection (ANC).

PHOSPHOLIPASE A2

Biochemical marker of necrotizing acute pancreatitis.

PIGTAIL

Pigtail drains are used for percutaneous catheter drainage (PCD) of **fluid collection** and **pseudocyst**.

PLANNED

In case **necrosectomy** is considered to be inadequate or incomplete in the first instance, abdomen may not be closed (only skin may be sutured) for planned staged relaparotomy to complete the necrosectomy. This approach is associated with higher risk of intestinal **fistula** and **incisional hernia**.

PLEURAL EFFUSION

Pleural effusion, more commonly on the left side (Figure P.4), is often present in patients with acute pancreatitis—this is because

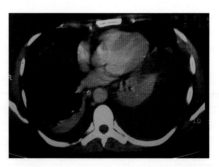

Figure P.4   Upper cuts of CT abdomen showing bilateral (left more than right) **pleural effusion** and consolidation in acute pancreatitis.

the tail of the pancreas lies close to the left dome of the diaphragm. It is also a risk predictor for severity and mortality.

PMN ELASTASE

Polymorphonuclear (PMN) elastase >120 ng/L indicates severe acute pancreatitis.

PNEUMONIA

Hospital-acquired pneumonia (HAP) and ventilator-associated pneumonia (VAP) are common in patients with severe acute pancreatitis.

POLYMERIC

Polymeric enteral diet is as good as an elemental diet with monosaccharides, amino acids, and short-chain fatty acids (SCFA).

POLYMORPHONUCLEAR ELASTASE

See **PMN elastase**

POP (PANCREATITIS OUTCOME PREDICTION)

Age, mean arterial pressure (MAP), urea, calcium, pH, PaO_2/FiO_2 are predictors of severity, necrosis, infection, local complications, MODS, and death in acute pancreatitis.

PORTEX

Wide bore (32–36 F) Portex tubes with multiple side holes are commonly used for drainage and **lavage** after surgical **necrosectomy**.

POST-ERCP ACUTE PANCREATITIS

See **ERCP-induced acute pancreatitis**

POSTOPERATIVE ACUTE PANCREATITIS

Operations on the pancreas itself (e.g., pancreatoduodenectomy), biliary tract (common bile duct [CBD] exploration), and the stomach and duodenum (distal gastrectomy) may result in postoperative acute pancreatitis which may be difficult to differentiate from the more common postoperative complications of these operations.

POSTPYLORIC FEEDING

Enteral feeding with a postpyloric (nasoduodenal or **nasojejunal**) tube is preferred to nasogastric feeding as it has less risk of aspiration of the feed.

PREDICTORS

Outcome of an attack of acute pancreatitis can be predicted using several host factors (e.g., age and BMI) and clinical factors (e.g., SIRS and response to initial therapy).

Old age (>55 years), **obesity** with high (>30) body mass index (BMI), alcoholic (cf. gallstones) etiology, high **APACHE** score, high (>45%) hematocrit (Hct), high CRP (>150), **organ failure** at onset of disease or early (within 7 days) in the course of the disease, **extent** of necrosis, and **infection** of **necrosis** are poor predictors of survival in acute pancreatitis.

Old **age** (>55 years), **obesity** with high (>30) body mass index (BMI), and **pleural effusion** are predictors of severity, infection, need for admission to HDU/ICU, and death in acute pancreatitis.

PRESERVATION

Preservation of viable pancreatic parenchyma is of utmost importance during **necrosectomy**. This is easier in patients who undergo a delayed operation (after 3rd or 4th week) because the necrotic process gets localized and there is clear demarcation between necrotic and viable parenchyma. In patients who are operated early (1st or 2nd week), the necrotic process may not have still localized (Figure P.5) and demarcation between necrotic and viable parenchyma may not be clear.

Too aggressive necrosectomy may remove viable pancreatic parenchyma, whereas too conservative necrosectomy may leave necrotic tissue behind.

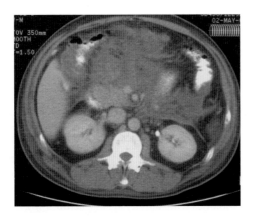

Figure P.5 Early necrosis—not yet well localized.

PREVALENCE

More than 200,000 admissions are done for acute pancreatitis in the USA every year.

PREVENTION

1. **Infection** of **necrosis** can be prevented by
   a. **Enteral nutrition**
   b. Selective gut decontamination (SGD)
   c. **Antibiotics**
2. Every attempt must be made to find out the **etiology** of acute pancreatitis in every patient so as to prevent its recurrence by correcting the cause, if possible.

PROBIOTICS

Use of probiotics is an attractive theoretical option but their routine use in acute pancreatitis needs more evidence.

PROCALCITONIN (PCT)

A marker of severity of acute pancreatitis, serum procalcitonin (PCT) >3.8 mg/mL is predictive of organ dysfunction in acute pancreatitis.

P

PROCEDURE INDUCED

Many diagnostic/therapeutic procedures (e.g., ERCP, endoscopic papillotomy [EPT], biliary manometry, EUS-guided FNAC of pancreas) can cause acute pancreatitis.

PROPHYLACTIC ANTIBIOTICS

The use of antibiotic prophylactic to prevent **infection** of **necrosis** is a matter of debate and controversy. Most metaanalyses conclude that prophylactic antibiotics are not effective, with no decrease in the risk of infection or mortality. Most groups, however, still use broad spectrum antibiotics with activity against aerobes and anaerobes in patients with severe acute pancreatitis (organ failure and necrosis).

PROPHYLACTIC STOMA

A prophylactic stoma (ileostomy) may be performed during operation for necrosectomy if the transverse colon is forming a part of the necrotic cavity.

PROTEASES

Enzymes causing inflammation in acute pancreatitis, e.g., TAP and leukocyte-derived PMN elastase.

PROTEASE INHIBITORS

Protease inhibitors such as **aprotinin** and **gabexate** have not been proved to be of benefit in acute pancreatitis.

PROTEOLYTIC ENZYMES

Ductal disruption leads to extravasation of the pancreatic juice containing proteolytic enzymes into the peripancreatic tissues.

PSEUDOANEURYSM

Pancreatic enzymes can erode into and weaken the wall of an adjacent artery and form a pseudoaneurysm. Commonest artery involved is the splenic artery followed by the gastroduodenal artery, middle colic artery, and the left gastric artery. Rupture of a pseudo-aneurysm into the pseudocyst results in sudden onset severe pain and increase in the size of the cyst. **Doppler** US is useful to detect a pseudoaneurysm; CT **angiography** is diagnostic (Figure P.6).

Conventional angiography shows extravasation of contrast (Figure P.7). Treatment of choice is **angioembolization** (Figure P.8).

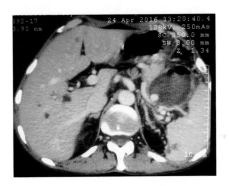

Figure P.6 CT angiogram showing an enhancing pseudoaneurysm in a pseudocyst.

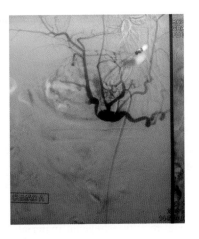

Figure P.7 Angiogram showing extravasation of contrast from the gastroduodenal artery.

P

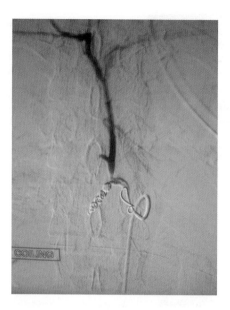

Figure P.8 Coil embolization of gastroduodenal artery.

PSEUDOCYST

Acute peripancreatic fluid collection (APFC) that persists beyond 4 weeks evolves into a pseudocyst. Revised Atlanta classification says pseudocysts are very rare in acute pancreatitis (but the author does not agree). Pseudocyst, one of the commonest delayed local complications of acute interstitial pancreatitis, is a well localized, circumscribed, peripancreatic collection of pancreatic amylase-rich fluid with no or minimal necrotic debris with a mature wall of inflammatory granulation and fibrous tissue (cf. **fluid collection**—no wall; cf. **abscess**—contains pus). Most pseudocysts form in the vicinity of pancreas, but they can occur at distant sites also.

US and CT show a well-defined, smooth cyst with anechoic fluid contents (Figure P.9); echogenic material (debris) may be present.

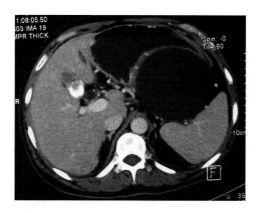

Figure P.9 CT showing **pseudocyst** behind the stomach which is compressed anteriorly.

Pseudocyst may form after pancreatic trauma and in chronic pancreatitis also.

Pseudocysts, following acute pancreatitis, even if large (>6 cm) or persisting for long (>6 weeks), may be managed conservatively if they are asymptomatic; most of them resolve on their own.

While an acute pseudocyst (following an attack of acute pancreatitis) may resolve spontaneously even if it is large, a chronic pseudocyst (in a patient with chronic pancreatitis) needs intervention.

Indications of intervention (surgical, endoscopic, or percutaneous) in a pseudocyst are:

1. Symptoms, e.g., pain, postprandial fullness, early satiety
2. Complications, e.g., infection (resulting in an **abscess**), bleeding, rupture, and obstruction of the CBD or the duodenum
3. Doubt of malignancy (**cystic tumor**)
4. Failure to resolve (increasing size or no decrease in size over a period of time)

It is called pseudocyst as it has a wall of granulation and fibrous tissue with no epithelial lining (cf. epithelial wall of a true cyst).

P

Adjacent organs, e.g., stomach (Figure P.9), form a part of the wall of the pseudocyst—hence, it cannot be excised (cf. true cyst). A pseudocyst may communicate with the pancreatic duct.

PULMONARY COMPLICATIONS

Patients with severe acute pancreatitis may develop several pulmonary complications, e.g., atelectasis, pneumonitis, pleural effusion, and ARDS, resulting in tachypnea, dyspnea, hypoxemia, and respiratory failure.

P

Q

QUINOLONES

Fluoroquinolones such as ciprofloxacin and ofloxacin have good penetration in pancreatic tissue and achieve high concentration in pancreatic parenchyma. They are therefore preferred in patients with acute pancreatitis as a cheaper option to more expensive **carbapenems**.

Q

R

RADIOLOGY

Radiology, for diagnosis of acute pancreatitis, includes CT or MRI (not US).

RANSON'S CRITERIA (1974)

At admission—age >55 years, WBC >16,000 mm^3, glucose >200 mg/dL, LDH >350 IU/L, and AST (SGOT) >250 U/L.

During 48 hours—Hct fall >10%, BUN rise >5 mg/dL, PaO$_2$ <60 mm Hg, base deficit >5 mEq, fluid sequestration >6 liters, and calcium <8 mg/dL.

A Ranson score of 3 or more indicates severe acute pancreatitis. Ranson score also predicts mortality; <3 (<1%), 3–4 (15%), 5–6 (40%), and >6 (100%).

The main disadvantage of using Ranson's criteria is that the assessment requires a mandatory 48 hours period.

RANSON'S CRITERIA, MODIFIED

Eleven criteria (age, hematocrit, WBC count, blood glucose, blood urea, serum albumin, AST, LDH, calcium, PaO$_2$, pH) assessed within 48 hours of admission.

READMISSION

Patients with acute pancreatitis may require readmission for:

1. A repeat attack of acute pancreatitis
2. Residual problems after an attack has apparently resolved

RECURRENT

1. Recurrent acute pancreatitis (RAP) is defined as two or more attacks of acute pancreatitis. The commonest cause is biliary stone disease, **sludge**, or **microlithiasis**; other causes include **hypercalceamia**, **hyperlipidemia**, **pancreas divisum**, **choledochocele**, **perivaterian diverticulum**, and **worms**. It can also occur in a background of **chronic pancreatitis** or pancreatic cancer. No etiology can be found in about one-third of patients with recurrent acute pancreatitis—**idiopathic**.
2. If the gall bladder is not removed, a significant number (one-fourth to two-thirds) of patients with biliary acute pancreatitis will have recurrence of acute pancreatitis.
3. Recurrent attacks of acute pancreatitis may cause a fibrotic stricture in the pancreatic duct and lead to chronic pancreatitis.

REFERRAL

Patients who are at high risk (see **Risk factors**, **Risk predictors**) and those with severe acute pancreatitis should be referred to a center where facilities and expertise for intensive care, interventional radiology, and therapeutic endoscopy are available.

REFLUX

Obstruction of the sphincter of **Oddi** and the ampulla of **Vater** can result in reflux of bile into the pancreatic duct causing acute pancreatitis.

REMOTE COLLECTIONS

Acute fluid collections are usually peripancreatic but may be remote (Figure R.1) from the pancreas, anywhere in the abdomen.

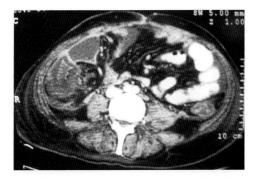

Figure R.1 Acute fluid collections remote from the pancreas.

REMOTE ORGANS

Toxins released during an attack of acute pancreatitis may affect remote organs, e.g., lungs, kidneys, heart, brain, and result in multiple organ dysfunction syndrome (MODS).

REOPERATION

Reoperations are not infrequently required for residual necrosis, residual fluid collection/sepsis, and bowel (usually colonic or jejunal) perforation and bleeding in patients who have undergone necrosectomy. Reoperation can be **planned**/scheduled if the necrosectomy is judged to be incomplete (more likely in patients who are operated early)—**laparostomy** (open abdomen) may be performed in such cases. Reoperation can be **on demand** (SOS), if the necrosectomy is judged to be complete (more likely in patients who are operated late)—abdomen is closed (with drains) in such cases.

REPEAT

1. Serum **amylase** and **lipase** levels should be repeated if they are normal initially but the suspicion of acute pancreatitis persists.
2. Criteria for assessment of **severity** may have to be repeated after a few days as severity of acute pancreatitis is a dynamic status.

3. Organ functions should be repeated as **transient** organ dysfunction does not carry as bad prognosis as **persisting** organ dysfunction.
4. Repeat CTs are often required in patients with acute pancreatitis to monitor the progress of fluid collections/necrosis and to look for complications.
5. Even if the initial US does not show gallstones (GS), a repeat US should be done at a later stage to reconfirm the absence of GS.

RESECTION

Although some surgeons use the term resection to describe the operative procedure—**necrosectomy** is a better term because only nonviable, devitalized, necrotic, sloughed, pancreatic, and peripancreatic tissues are removed (by finger, blunt dissection, suction) rather than resection by formal sharp dissection.

RESIDUAL

Residual necrosis/infection is very common after **necrosectomy**, especially if necrosectomy was done early during the phase of acute pancreatitis. Fever, tachycardia, dyspnea, unsettled abdomen, and persisting or worsening organ function are clinical indicators; CT is confirmatory. Majority of residual infections can be drained percutaneously; some (no safe access, multiple fluid collections, multiloculated fluid collections, solid necrotic debris) may require surgical drainage.

RESOURCE INTENSIVE

Management of acute pancreatitis is a highly resource-intensive affair, resulting in very high cost burden to the family, hospital, and the society.

RESPONSE

Response to conservative management should be closely monitored; failure to respond/deterioration is an indication for imaging and/or intervention.

REST

It was thought that pancreas should be "rested" by stopping enteral feeds completely. It is, however, now established that this is not true, and enteral feeding is not only harmless but may be beneficial in acute pancreatitis.

RESUSCITATION

Mainstay of resuscitation in acute pancreatitis is early adequate fluid replacement.

Patients with acute pancreatitis may need large-volume (6–8 L/day) fluid resuscitation.

RETCHING

Retching, along with nausea and vomiting, is very frequent in acute pancreatitis.

RETROCOLIC

Collections (Figure R.2) and necrosis (Figure R.3) may extend into the retrocolic retroperitoneal tissue—more commonly on the left side.

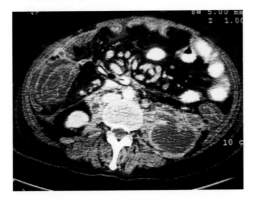

R

Figure R.2 Retrocolic collection on the left side; there is subparietal collection on the right side also.

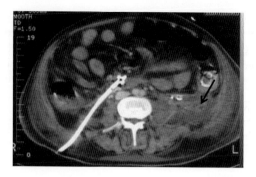

Figure R.3 **Retrocolic** necrosis (arrow) on the left side.

RETROPERITONEAL APPROACH

Retroperitoneal approach through a left lateral flank incision (Figure R.4) anterior to and below the 12th rib between the left kidney and the descending colon provides good access to the lesser sac without contaminating the main peritoneal cavity. This approach may not, however, provide adequate access to the head of the pancreas and the right retrocolic space. It is also

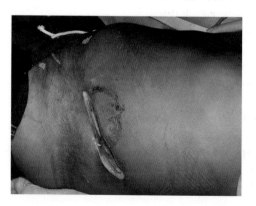

Figure R.4 Left flank incision for **retroperitoneal** necrosectomy.

not recommended in patients with extensive infracolic, mesenteric, and retroperitoneal necrosis where a midline laparotomy is better. Obviously, a simultaneous cholecystectomy cannot be performed.

RINGER'S LACTATE

Ringer's lactate is preferred as the IV fluid of choice for initial resuscitation in acute pancreatitis; it may be associated with less risk of SIRS than normal saline.

RISK FACTORS

Obesity, high **APACHE** score, shock (BP <80 mm Hg), and renal or pulmonary dysfunction are the risk factors for mortality in patients with severe acute pancreatitis.

RISK IDENTIFICATION

From among patients with acute pancreatitis, it is important to identify those who have or are at risk to have severe acute pancreatitis as they need intensive management in HDU/ICU. Several scores/indices, e.g., **Ranson**, **Balthazar**, **Glasgow (Imrie)**, have been used for this risk identification.

R

ROOF TOP

Bilateral subcostal incision for **necrosectomy**—especially in obese, heavy built patients with a wide costal margin.

RUPTURE

A **pseudocyst** may rupture into the gastrointestinal (GI) tract, resulting in GI **bleed** and spontaneous resolution of the cyst. An US should, therefore, always be obtained on the day prior to intervention in every patient with a pseudocyst.

RYLE'S TUBE

Ryle's (nasogastric) tube aspiration and drainage of the stomach is indicated in patients with persistent vomiting. It also helps in decreasing pancreatic stimulation and secretion by preventing acidic gastric juice entering the duodenum.

R

S

SANTORINI, DUCT OF

Dorsal (minor) pancreatic duct, which normally drains only the superior half of the head of the pancreas; in pancreas divisum, the duct of Santorini assumes importance because it has to drain the superior half of the head, body, and tail of the pancreas.

SaO$_2$

Arterial saturation of oxygen (also **SpO$_2$**); normal 100%.

SAPONIFICATION

Pancreatic juice results in saponification of retroperitoneal and omental fat—saponification utilizes calcium, resulting in **hypocalcaemia** of acute pancreatitis.

SATURATION

Arterial oxygen saturation (**SaO$_2$**) must be monitored—arterial blood gas (ABG) analysis should be done if SaO$_2$ is <95%.

SCORES

Several prognostic scores have been described for acute pancreatitis. They could be one time (e.g., **APACHE II**) or over a period of time (e.g., **Ranson**).

SCORPION

Scorpion sting can cause acute pancreatitis.

SDD (SELECTIVE DECONTAMINATION OF THE DIGESTIVE TRACT)

See **Selective gut decontamination**

SECRETIN

Secretin-induced MRCP better delineates the pancreatic duct.

SECOND HIT

An untimely surgical intervention may act as a second hit (following the first hit of the disease) and result in deterioration of the patient's condition.

SELECTIVE GUT DECONTAMINATION (SGD)

Translocation of bacteria across the inflamed gut (colonic) wall is an important cause of infection of peripancreatic **fluid collections/necrosis**. Some groups use SGD with oral nonabsorbable antibiotics, such as neomycin, to reduce this risk of **infection** of **necrosis** by decreasing bacterial **translocation** across the inflamed colonic wall.

SEMIOPEN METHOD

See **Closed laparostoma**

SENTINEL LOOP

Supine abdomen X-ray may reveal a dilated proximal jejunal loop in the left upper abdomen due to localized inflammatory paralytic ileus.

SEPSIS

Infection of peripancreatic fluid collection and infection of necrosis cause sepsis and septic complications in the later phase (2nd and 3rd week) of acute pancreatitis. Source of sepsis may, however, be catheters (central venous, urinary) or tubes (endotracheal).

SEPTATE

In a pseudocyst with multiple septae, a **cystic neoplasm** of the pancreas should be suspected. EUS-guided aspiration of fluid and its analysis for amylase, CEA, CA 19-9, and fluid cytology helps.

SEPTIC COMPLICATIONS

A large number of patients with acute pancreatitis, especially those who undergo intervention, suffer from septic complications.

SEQUELAE

It was originally thought that acute pancreatitis does not result in any long-term anatomical damage to the gland or the duct. An attack of acute pancreatitis may, however, cause fibrotic stricture of the pancreatic duct leading to **chronic pancreatitis**. Extensive pancreatic necrosis may result in endocrine (diabetes) and exocrine (steatorrhea) insufficiency.

SEQUESTRATION

A large volume of fluid can sequestrate in the inflamed peripancreatic retroperitoneal space, resulting in hypovolemia requiring replacement with liters of fluid.

S

SEVERE

Once a diagnosis of acute pancreatitis has been made, the most important issue is to classify the severity of the attack; this is important for planning the management and for predicting the outcome. Clinical features are poor markers for assessment of severity of acute pancreatitis, and severity of pain does not indicate severity of acute pancreatitis. Similarly, levels of serum **amylase/lipase** do not correlate with the severity of acute pancreatitis.

Hct, CRP, TAP, and **PMN elastase** are stand-alone markers for severity of acute pancreatitis.

Local complications, e.g., **fluid collection**, **pseudocyst**, and/or presence of multiple organ dysfunction syndrome (MODS), classify an attack of acute pancreatitis as severe.

Presence of **necrosis** on contrast-enhanced CT also indicates severe acute pancreatitis.

About 15%–20% of patients with acute pancreatitis have severe disease. Mortality of severe acute pancreatitis may be as high as 25%–30%.

SEVERITY

Severity of an attack of acute pancreatitis may range from mild (self-limiting lasting for a few days) through moderately severe to severe (resulting in MODS and death).

SGD

See **Selective gut decontamination**

SHARP DISSECTION

Sharp dissection, e.g., with scissors, should be avoided during **necrosectomy** as it may cause bleeding; **blunt** dissection, e.g., with finger, suction tip, or sponge holder, is preferred.

SHOCK

Patients with severe acute pancreatitis may present to the A&E in shock and may be misdiagnosed as a cardiac patient.

SIGNS

Abdominal signs are usually less than the symptoms in patients with acute pancreatitis. These include distension, tenderness, and guarding in the upper abdomen; bowel sounds may be absent.

SILICONIZED

Siliconized drains are preferred for drainage and **lavage** after **necrosectomy** as they may have to be retained for long. PVC tubes tend to get stiffened and may erode into adjacent viscera/vessels.

SIMV

Synchronized (effort triggered) intermittent mandatory ventilation—ventilation is assisted at the time of spontaneous inspiration. SIMV mode is often used to wean the patient off from intermittent positive pressure ventilation (IPPV).

SINUSITIS

Patients with prolonged (>2 weeks) insertion of a nasal (nasogastric/nasoduodenal/nasojejunal) tube have a high risk of developing infection of the paranasal sinuses.

SIPS

While the patient is kept nil by mouth, few sips of water can safely be allowed.

SIRS (SYSTEMIC INFLAMMATORY RESPONSE SYNDROME)

Activation of inflammatory **cytokines** causes SIRS in the first 2 weeks of acute pancreatitis.

S

Presence of two or more of the following criteria confirms the presence of SIRS:

1. Pulse rate >90 beats/min
2. Respiratory rate >20/min or PCO_2 <32 mm Hg
3. Rectal temperature <36°C or >38°C
4. White blood cell count <4000 or >12,000/mm^3 or presence of bands >10%
5. Early onset and persistent SIRS in acute pancreatitis predicts high mortality

SIZE

Size >6 cm of an acute **pseudocyst** was earlier considered to be an indication for intervention. This is no longer true. Even large (>6 cm) acute pseudocysts can be observed provided they are asymptomatic and have no complications. As many as one-third of pseudocysts that are >6 cm in diameter may resolve on their own (cf. 2/3rd which are <6 cm).

Severe pain with sudden increase in size of a preexisting pseudocyst suggests an intracystic bleed (Figures S.1 and S.2).

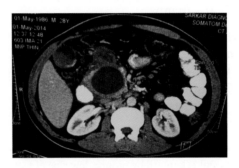

Figure S.1 Pseudocyst (May 1, 2014) with clear fluid.

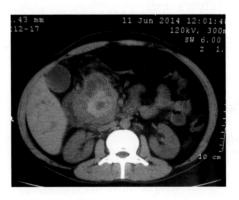

Figure S.2 Same patient (June 11, 2014) after an attack of severe pain and sudden increase in size of the palpable lump; CT showing hyperdense blood.

S

SLUDGE, BILIARY

Crystals of cholesterol and calcium bilirubinate in bile can cause acute pancreatitis. They can be seen on microscopic examination of duodenal bile.

SNAKE BITE

Snake bite can cause acute pancreatitis.

SOCIETIES

Several scientific societies, viz., American Gastroenterology Association (AGA), American Pancreatic Society (APS), European Pancreatic Club (EPC), International Association of Pancreatology (IAP), and Pancreatic Club and Society for Surgery of the Alimentary Tract (SSAT), contributed to and supported the revised Atlanta classification of acute pancreatitis.

SOFA (SEQUENTIAL ORGAN FAILURE ASSESSMENT)

SOFA >4 at 48 hours predicts severe acute pancreatitis.

SOOD (SPHINCTER OF ODDI DYSFUNCTION)

S

Sphincter of **Oddi** dysfunction (due to stenosis, fibrosis, or dyskinesia, resulting in increased [>40 mm Hg; normal being 15 mm Hg] pressure of the sphincter) may be the cause of acute pancreatitis/**recurrent** acute pancreatitis. It can be diagnosed by biliary/pancreatic manometry and is treated by endoscopic sphincterotomy.

SPECIFIC

Unfortunately, there is no specific treatment of acute pancreatitis. All treatments are only supportive.

SPECTRUM

The clinical spectrum of acute pancreatitis ranges from a mild, self-limiting attack (which may even remain undiagnosed or misdiagnosed as upper abdominal dyspepsia) to a severe rapidly progressive attack leading to MODS and death.

SPHINCTER OF ODDI

See **Oddi, Sphincter of**

SPLANCHNIC

Splanchnic vasoconstriction caused by inflammatory mediators released during an attack of acute pancreatitis may result in gut mucosal ischemia.

SPLENIC VEIN THROMBOSIS (SVT)

Peripancreatic inflammation may lead to SVT and left-sided portal hypertension with splenomegaly and gastric varices causing upper GI bleed. If the splenic vein thrombosis and portal hypertension are of some duration, collaterals (Figure S.3) may be present which can bleed profusely during necrosectomy.

Most SVT will resolve with recanalization of the splenic vein after acute pancreatitis has settled. If SVT and portal hypertension persist, splenectomy may be required.

A pseudocyst may also cause compression of the splenic vein and splenomegaly (Figure S.4).

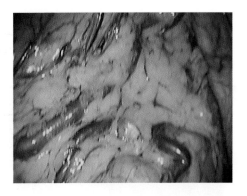

Figure S.3 Collaterals in the gastrocolic omentum due to portal hypertension caused by splenic vein thrombosis in acute pancreatitis.

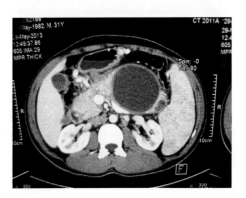

Figure S.4 Compression of the splenic vein and splenomegaly caused by a pseudocyst.

SpO₂

Arterial oxygen saturation (also **SaO₂**).

SPONGE HOLDER

A sponge holder (Figure S.5) is a good instrument to remove the necrotic debris during surgical **necrosectomy**.

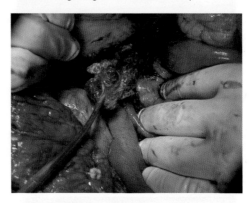

Figure S.5 Sponge holder being used to remove solid necrotic debris.

STARVATION

Prolonged starvation of patients with acute pancreatitis is not recommended. Nil-by-mouth policy is recommended only in the first few days of an attack of acute pancreatitis when the patient may be hemodynamically unstable or has paralytic ileus. Oral/enteral feeds should be introduced as soon as possible—usually within few days.

STEATORRHEA

Patients with extensive pancreatic **necrosis/necrosectomy** may develop exocrine insufficiency, manifesting as steatorrhea (large volume, bulky, frothy foul-smelling stools), in the long term.

STEP-UP APPROACH

Initial conservative management followed by nonsurgical (percutaneous, radiological, and endoscopic) intervention or minimally invasive (laparoscopic) surgical intervention if required—laparotomy is a final resort only. Intervention should preferably be retro (extra) peritoneal first, followed by transluminal (endoscopic) and transperitoneal.

STERILE NECROSIS

Sterile necrosis is treated conservatively; progressive deterioration in the overall organ functional status may, however, indicate intervention even for sterile necrosis.

STOMACH

A pseudocyst in the lesser sac lies in close proximity to the posterior wall of the stomach (Figure S.6) and is eminently suitable for endoscopic drainage into the stomach.

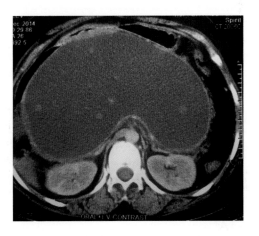

Figure S.6 Pseudocyst in close proximity to the posterior wall of the stomach.

STRANDING

Peripancreatic (Figure S.7), mesenteric, retroperitoneal, perirenal, and retrocolic fat stranding (indicating inflammation) is a very common CT finding in acute pancreatitis.

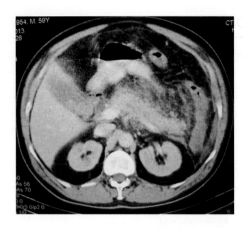

Figure S.7 Peripancreatic fat stranding in acute pancreatitis.

STREPTOKINASE

Streptokinase may be used to lyse necrotic debris after percutaneous catheter drainage (PCD) of ANC or WON to ensure its better removal.

STRESS ULCER

Patients with severe acute pancreatitis can have upper gastrointestinal (GI) bleed from stress ulcers in the stomach and should receive prophylaxis with H_2 receptor antagonists (H_2RAs) or proton pump inhibitors (PPIs).

SUBCOSTAL

Bilateral subcostal (**roof top**) incision for **necrosectomy** in short, stout individuals with a wide costal margin and in patients with predominantly lesser sac (supracolic) necrosis.

SUCRALFATE

Sucralfate, a mucosal coating agent, protects the stomach against **stress ulcers** and decreases the risk of aspiration pneumonia.

SUCTION TIP

A blunt suction tip (Figure S.8) can be used to suck out pus and pieces of necrotic solid debris during necrosectomy.

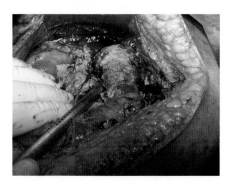

Figure S.8 Blunt suction tip being used during necrosectomy.

SUDDEN

1. Onset of pain in acute pancreatitis is usually sudden, as in **perforated peptic ulcer**, leaking or ruptured abdominal aortic aneurysm (AAA), **aortic dissection**, acute mesenteric ischemia (AMI), etc. It is, therefore, very important to exclude these surgically correctable conditions before a diagnosis of acute pancreatitis is made.
2. Sudden increase in the size of a **pseudocyst** (with pain) indicates an intracystic bleed.

SUPPURATIVE PANCREATITIS

A term used in the earlier classification—not used now.

SURFACE ANATOMY

The head of the pancreas overlies L1 and L2; body of the pancreas extends upward to the left; tail of the pancreas lies in the splenic hilum at T12 level. In a CT scan, therefore, the tail of the pancreas is seen first (cranial) followed by the body and then the head (caudal).

SURGICAL ACUTE ABDOMEN

Before a diagnosis of acute pancreatitis is made, surgical causes of **acute abdomen**, **perforated peptic ulcer**, acute mesenteric ischemia (AMI), and leaking/ruptured abdominal aortic aneurysm (AAA) should be excluded—this may require an early (on admission) CT.

SURGICAL COMPLICATIONS

Complications such as bleed, bowel gangrene, perforation, and fistula may indicate surgical intervention in acute pancreatitis. Patients with abdominal compartment syndrome (ACS) may benefit from abdominal decompression.

SURGICAL INTERVENTION

Surgical intervention may be required in patients with acute pancreatitis for:

1. Management of **necrosis** (especially **infected**)
2. Management of **surgical complications**
3. Prevention of **recurrent** acute pancreatitis

SUSPICION

Infection should be suspected in pancreatic necrosis if the clinical condition of a patient with severe acute pancreatitis worsens in spite of **organ support**.

SUSTAINED

Sustained (cf. **transient**, reversible) organ failure is a strong predictor of mortality—as high as one out of three patients with sustained organ failure will die.

SVT

See **Splenic vein thrombosis**

SWAN GANZ

A Swan-Ganz catheter monitors the pulmonary arterial pressure. This may be better than monitoring the central venous pressure (CVP) only, especially in patients with severe cardiac and respiratory disease.

SYSTEMIC COMPLICATIONS

Cardiovascular—systolic BP <90 mm Hg
Respiratory—arterial PaO_2 <60 mm Hg
Renal—serum creatinine >2 mg/dL
Coagulation (DIC)—platelets <100,000/dL, fibrinogen <1g/L, FDP >80 µg/mL
Metabolic—hypocalcaemia with calcium <7.5 mg/dL

S

T

TACHYCARDIA

A manifestation of systemic inflammatory response syndrome (SIRS).

TACHYPNEA

A manifestation of systemic inflammatory response syndrome (SIRS).

TAP (TRYPSINOGEN-ACTIVATION PEPTIDE)

Urinary trypsinogen-activation peptide TAP (done as a bedside dipstick test) is a marker of severity of acute pancreatitis.

TEAM

Patients with severe acute pancreatitis should preferably be managed by a team of gastroenterologists, endoscopists, radiologists, intensivists, and surgeons.

TEMPORIZATION

Percutaneous radiological intervention in the form of needle aspiration or catheter drainage may buy time before surgical intervention in patients with infected fluid collection/necrosis.

TEN

Transluminal (transgastric) endoscopic necrosectomy—multiple sessions are usually required.

TERMS

Several terms used in relation to acute pancreatitis have imprecise and confusing meanings. Atlanta classifications (both original and revised) have attempted to standardize these terms.

TETANY

Clinical tetany may occur as a result of severe **hypocalcaemia** in severe acute pancreatitis.

THIRD SPACE

Large volumes of plasma may extravasate into the extravascular third space in the retroperitoneum and elsewhere.

THROMBOCYTOPENIA

Thrombocytopenia is not uncommon in patients with severe acute pancreatitis and is a predictor of poor prognosis.

THROMBOSIS

The incidence of **splenic vein thrombosis** and portal vein thrombosis in acute pancreatitis is less than that in chronic pancreatitis. The resultant portal hypertension and esophagogastric varices cause upper gastrointestinal bleeding. **Doppler** US is diagnostic. Bleeding varies need endoscopic management.

TIME

1. Four weeks is the conventional watershed between acute **fluid collection** versus **pseudocyst** and **necrosis** versus **abscess**. It is, however, important to keep in mind that in a good number of cases, a fluid collection may not evolve into a pseudocyst and necrosis may not localize into an abscess even after 4 weeks.
2. **Infection** of **necrosis** is time dependent—about 25% in the 1st week, 35% in the 2nd week, and as high as 70% in the 3rd week.

TIMING OF CHOLECYSTECTOMY

In patients with mild acute pancreatitis, cholecystectomy should be performed in the same hospital admission (within 14 days) to prevent another attack of acute pancreatitis.

In patients with severe acute pancreatitis, cholecystectomy may have to be delayed for 4–6 weeks after the attack has settled to allow the inflammation to subside.

TIMING OF CT

CT should be performed in acute pancreatitis preferably after 72–96 hours of onset of attack so that the complete extent and degree of necrosis, if any, is evaluated. (The author prefers to obtain the first CT after 5–7 days.)

An **early** CT may be required in patients with undiagnosed **acute** (upper) **abdomen** to make the correct diagnosis of acute pancreatitis and, more importantly, to rule out surgical causes, e.g., perforated peptic ulcer, leaking/ruptured abdominal aortic aneurysm (AAA), and acute mesenteric ischemia (AMI), due to superior mesenteric vein thrombosis (Figure T.1).

Repeat CT is indicated if a patient with acute pancreatitis does not show expected improvement or deteriorates in spite of **organ support**.

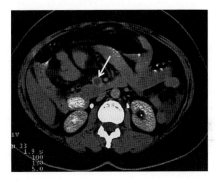

Figure T.1 Early CT showing superior mesenteric vein thrombosis (arrow) in a patient who was diagnosed clinically as acute pancreatitis.

TIMING OF DETECTION OF NECROSIS

Necrosis cannot be detected in the first 48 hours of onset; it is usually detectable between 2 and 7 days of onset when the first CT should be done.

TIMING OF FNA

There is not much point in doing FNA before 2 weeks because even if it is positive no surgery will be done; in the first 2 weeks, acute pancreatitis, by and large, is a "medical" disease.

TIMING OF INFECTIONS

NPIs (nonpancreatic infections) occur in the first 2 weeks, while IPN (infected pancreatic necrosis) is common during 3–4 weeks.

TIMING OF SURGERY

More and more groups now believe that the management of acute pancreatitis in its early phase (first 2 weeks) is largely medical; nonsurgical (radiological or endoscopic) intervention may be required in some cases. Surgical intervention should be delayed as far as possible—preferably beyond 4 weeks (certainly beyond 2–3 weeks). Delayed surgical intervention is associated with less mortality than early surgical intervention.

TOTAL PARENTERAL NUTRITION (TPN)

See **Parenteral nutrition**

TOXINS

A large number of toxic substances such as **trypsinogen**, trypsinogen-activation peptide (TAP), phospholipase A2, and polymorphonuclear (PMN) **elastase** are released during an attack of acute pancreatitis.

TPN (TOTAL PARENTERAL NUTRITION)

See **Parenteral nutrition**

TRACHEOSTOMY

Patients with severe acute pancreatitis and adult respiratory distress syndrome (ARDS) who could require prolonged ventilation may be better off with a tracheostomy. This reduces the dead space and improves tracheobronchial toilet.

Tracheostomy, however, is a common cause of nosocomial hospital-acquired pneumonia (HAP).

TRANSGASTRIC

Endoscopic transgastric **drainage** of a pseudocyst should preferably be performed under endoscopic ultrasonography (EUS) guidance which delineates approximation of the stomach and the cyst walls and ensures absence of any major vessels at the site of the puncture. **Endoscopic drainage** gives better results in pseudocysts with all fluid content and no solid necrotic debris.

A transgastric percutaneous catheter drainage (PCD) (Figure T.2) may be required to externally drain a retrogastric fluid collection or abscess.

Endoscopic transgastric necrosectomy has also been reported. See **TEN**.

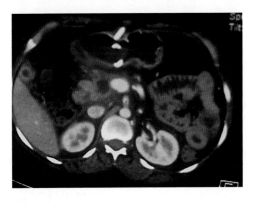

Figure T.2 Transgastric percutaneous catheter drain (PCD) in situ.

TRANSIENT

Transient, i.e., <48 hours (cf. **persistent**, i.e., >48 hours) organ failure may be present in moderately severe acute pancreatitis.

TRANSLOCATION

Mucosal ischemia due to hypotension and increased permeability of the gut wall due to inflammation are responsible for translocation of enteric bacteria from the gut lumen across the bowel wall, resulting in **infection** of peripancreatic **fluid collection** and **necrosis**.

Bacterial translocation can be prevented/reduced by instituting **enteral nutrition**.

TRAUMA

Abdominal trauma is the commonest cause of acute pancreatitis in children. Both blunt and penetrating trauma can cause acute pancreatitis due to ductal disruption, leading to leakage and collection of the pancreatic juice (Figure T.3).

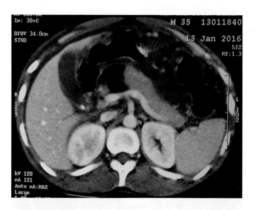

Figure T.3 Pancreatic **trauma** with transection of the gland and peripancreatic fluid collection.

TRYPSIN

Activation of trypsin is one of the first steps in the pathophysiology of acute pancreatitis. Trypsin inhibitors, e.g., **aprotinin,** however, have not been found to be useful in the management of acute pancreatitis.

TRYPSINOGEN

Inactive trypsinogen gets converted to active **trypsin**, a protease which is responsible for the autodigestion of tissues in acute pancreatitis. Urinary trypsinogen dipstick is a rapid noninvasive bedside test to diagnose acute pancreatitis.

TRYPSINOGEN ACTIVATION PEPTIDE

See **TAP**

TUMOR

Periampullary (Figure T.4) or pancreatic head tumors including adenocarcinoma, neuroendocrine tumors (NET), cystic tumors, intraductal papillary mucinous tumors (IPMN), etc., may obstruct the pancreatic duct and present as acute pancreatitis.

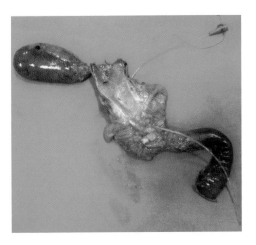

Figure T.4 This patient had an episode of acute pancreatitis; US did not show any gallstones but CBD was dilated till its lower end. Side-viewing endoscopy showed a papillary periampullary tumor; CT showed a resectable lesion and pancreatoduodenectomy was done.

T

U

UDCA (URSODEOXYCHOLIC ACID)

One of the options of management in patients with **microlithiasis** is ursodeoxycholic acid UDCA (10 mg/Kg/day in divided doses).

UNCERTAIN

Uncertain diagnosis in an acute abdomen is an indication for early CT at admission.

UNPREDICTABLE

Patients with acute pancreatitis (especially severe acute pancreatitis) have a highly unpredictable course and, therefore, need to be very closely monitored for any deterioration.

UNWELLNESS

Persistent unwellness (failure to thrive) suggests infection of necrosis and may indicate intervention.

UP SIZE

The PCD (percutaneous catheter drain) site is gradually dilated, and drains are serially up sized for better evacuation of necrotic debris.

URINE OUTPUT

A urine output of 0.5–1.0 mL/Kg/hour should be targeted while the patient is being hydrated.

US (ULTRASONOGRAPHY)

US is a poor investigation for evaluation of the pancreas, more so in presence of obesity, gaseous distention, and paralytic ileus. US would, however, be done in majority of patients with acute pancreatitis not to make its diagnosis but to rule out other diagnoses as the clinical diagnosis is of **acute** (upper) **abdomen**. US is not a useful investigation for the diagnosis of **necrosis** and for evaluation of the extent of necrosis—contrast-enhanced CT is the investigation of choice for this purpose. Altered heterogeneous echotexture of a bulky pancreas indicates inflammation but a normal pancreas on US does not rule out (mild) acute pancreatitis. US is, however, a good investigation for evaluation of the biliary tract (gallstones, intrahepatic biliary radical dilatation [IHBRD], dilated common bile duct [CBD], and **CBD** stone [Figure U.1], peripancreatic **fluid collection**, and **pleural effusion**).

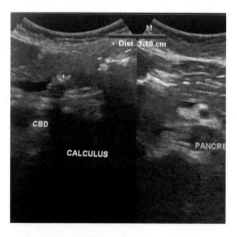

Figure U.1 US showing CBD stone.

In a patient with acute pancreatitis, if the initial US is negative for GS, it should be repeated at least once at a later date to confirm the absence of GS.

US is also a useful tool during follow-up of a patient with acute pancreatitis to detect **pseudocyst** (smooth walls with anechoic contents).

It is also used to monitor the progress of a pseudocyst which is being observed. It can detect bleed in a pseudocyst (Figure U.2).

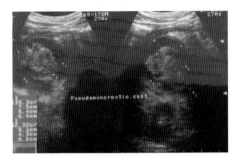

Figure U.2 US showing bleed in a pseudocyst seen as hyper-echoic contents.

US is also used for image-guided diagnostic and therapeutic interventions, e.g., fine-needle aspiration (FNA), for diagnosis of infection in a fluid collection or necrosis, needle aspiration, and percutaneous catheter drainage (PCD) of fluid collection or ascites.

US can also detect **air** in necrosis (to indicate infection) and can differentiate between fluid and solid necrotic debris in a pseudocyst.

UTI (URINARY TRACT INFECTION)

Almost all patients with severe acute pancreatitis require to be catheterized at some stage or the other and are at risk to develop urinary tract infection (UTI), especially with **nosocomial** organisms.

U

V

VARD

Video-assisted retroperitoneal debridement (VARD) through a small **retroperitoneal** flank incision using a **nephroscope**.

VASCULITIS

Vasculitides, e.g., systemic lupus erythematosus (SLE) and poly-arteritis nodosa (PAN), can cause acute pancreatitis.

VASCULAR COMPLICATIONS

Vascular complications of acute pancreatitis include **splenic vein thrombosis** and arterial **pseudoaneurysm** of adjacent vessels.

VASOACTIVE SUBSTANCES

Several vasoactive substances produced by the inflamed and necrotic pancreas are responsible for the remote organ dysfunction/failure.

VASOPRESSORS

Vasopressors such as dopamine, dobutamine, adrenaline, nor-adrenaline are useful in patients with hypotension and shock but should be administered only after fluid has been adequately replaced and central venous pressure (CVP) has been restored.

VENOMOUS

Inflamed pancreas is a venomous snake which is best left untouched. Even a snake charmer should try to catch it only if he is sure to catch it.

VENOUS BLOOD

A mixed venous blood sample is easier to obtain than arterial for frequent monitoring of oxygenation—SaO_2 of venous blood is 70% (cf. 100% in arterial blood) and PaO_2 is 40 mm (cf. 100 mm in arterial blood) Hg.

VENOUS THROMBOEMBOLISM (VTE)

Patients with severe acute pancreatitis who require prolonged admission to HDU/ICU are prone to develop venous thromboembolism (VTE)—deep venous thrombosis (DVT) (Figure V.1) and pulmonary embolism (PE)—and should be considered for VTE prophylaxis, both mechanical and pharmacological.

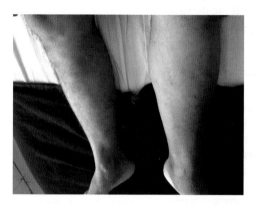

Figure V.1 Unilateral (left) leg edema in **deep venous thrombosis**.

VENTILATORY SUPPORT

Ventilatory support is an essential and important component of **organ support** in patients with organ dysfunction/failure.

VESSELS

Vessels, e.g., middle colic, are often appreciated (seen or felt) as a linear pulsatile structure bridging across the necrotic cavity in the lesser sac. Caution should be exercised during necrosectomy not to injure them.

VIDEO

VARD or necrosectomy through an extraperitoneal approach.

VIRAL

Several viral **infections**, e.g., mumps, cytomegalovirus (CMV), varicella zoster, and coxsackie, can cause acute pancreatitis.

VITAL SIGNS

Patients with acute pancreatitis usually have fever, tachycardia, and tachypnea; vital signs must be closely monitored.

VOLUME

1. Most patients require about 2500–4000 mL of fluids in the first 24 hours of resuscitation.
2. Management of patients with acute pancreatitis in a high volume (>100 patients/year) center is associated with decreased hospital stay and mortality.

VOMITING

Pain of acute pancreatitis is invariably associated with **nausea** and vomiting; vomiting in acute pancreatitis is, however, not copious and persistent, is not feculent and does not relieve pain (cf. intestinal obstruction).

W

WALLED-OFF NECROSIS (WON)

After a variable period of time (usually 4 or more weeks), an acute necrotic collection (ANC) may get well demarcated from the surrounding tissues and even assume a mature well-defined wall to form a localized encapsulated collection of solid necrotic debris (Figure W.1) with some (minimal) fluid (cf. pseudocyst which contains liquid with some [minimal] solid debris).

WON is usually peripancreatic but may be pancreatic also; multiple cavities are sometimes present (Figure W.2). WON may be sterile or infected. Many (sterile) WON may resolve on their own but infected WON will invariably require intervention. Sterile WON may require intervention if it persists say beyond 4–8 weeks with symptoms (e.g., pain, feeling of being unwell) or complications (e.g., gastric outlet obstruction, biliary obstruction, intestinal obstruction). Unlike a pseudocyst, WON may not be amenable to endoscopic drainage and may necessitate surgical evacuation.

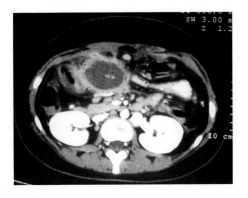

Figure W.1 Walled-off necrosis (WON) containing solid necrotic debris.

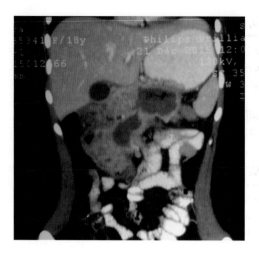

Figure W.2 Walled-off necrosis—two cavities.

WIDE

Clinical spectrum of acute pancreatitis is very wide—ranging from mild upper abdominal pain (which may be dismissed as gastritis) to very early multiorgan failure and death.

WINDOW

The first 48–72 hours from the onset of attack of acute pancreatitis is the window of opportunity for appropriate initial management, especially fluid replacement.

WIRSUNG, DUCT OF

The ventral (main) pancreatic duct which drains the lower part of the head of the pancreas and the uncinate process and the body and tail of the pancreas.

WON

See **Walled-off necrosis**

W

WORD, LAST

"The last 2 decades have taught the pancreatologists that many of our concepts of acute pancreatitis were naïve and even incorrect" (Sarr et al. 2013).

> *Shall we be saying the same thing in 2033 too?*
> *Last word on acute pancreatitis is yet to be written!*

WORMS

Intestinal worms, e.g., **ascaris**, clonorchis, liver fluke, can enter the pancreatic duct through the papilla and can cause acute pancreatitis.

WOUND

Wound infection and dehiscence are very frequent after surgery for pancreatic necrosis. Interrupted closure of the sheath/linea/aponeurosis is, therefore, recommended. Skin and subcutaneous tissues are approximated with a few far-placed interrupted sutures, or else a corrugated drain can be left in the subcutaneous plane.

Closure of the abdomen is usually difficult in patients with acute pancreatitis. This is because of retroperitoneal, bowel wall, and abdominal wall edema and ascites.

W

X

XANTHOMAS

May be seen around the eyes in patients with acute pancreatitis due to **hypertriglyceridemia**.

XIGRIS®

Human recombinant activated protein C which modifies the inflammatory and coagulation cascades—has not been proven of much role in acute pancreatitis.

X

Y

YEAST

Patients on long duration broad spectrum **antibiotics** are prone to get fungal infection with yeast.

YOUNG

CT should be used sparingly in young patients—MRI may be preferred.

Y

Z

ZIPPER

A zipper may be sutured to the edges of the wound of a laparotomy for **planned**/scheduled staged reexplorations—closed **laparostoma** or **semiopen** method.

ZYMOGEN

Pancreatic enzymes are stored as inactive zymogens granules. They are normally activated in the duodenum by enterokinase and activated **trypsinogen**.

Z

Suggested readings

BOOKS

Beger HG, Matsuno S, Cameron JL, eds. *Diseases of the Pancreas: Current Surgical Therapy*. Heidelberg, Germany: Springer, 2008 (Section 4 Acute pancreatitis).

Beger HG, Warshaw AL, Buchler MW, et al. *The Pancreas*. Oxford,MA: Blackwell, 2008 (Section 3 Acute pancreatitis).

Bhansali SK, Shah SC, eds. *Management of Acute Pancreatitis*. Mumbai: Jaslok Hospital, 2006.

Büchler M, Uhl W, Malfertheiner P, Sarr MG, eds. *Diseases of the Pancreas*. Basel, Switzerland: Karger, 2004.

Carter D, Russell RCG, Pitt HA, Bismuth H. *Rob & Smith's Operative Surgery. HepatoBiliary and Pancreatic Surgery*. London: Chapman & Hall Medical, 1998.

BOOK CHAPTERS

Sood S, Tandon V. Acute pancreatitis. In: Tandon BN, ed. *Tropical Hepatogastroenterology*. New Delhi: Elsevier, 2008: 539–565.

Subhalal N. Surgical treatment of acute pancreatitis. In: Chattopadhyay TK, ed. *GI Surgery Annual*, Vol 9. New Delhi: Indian Association of Surgical Gastroenterology, 2002: 35–50.

Thomas E Clancy, Stanley W Ashley. Management of acute pancreatitis. In: Zinner MJ, Stanley W Ashley, eds. Maingot's Abdominal Operations. New York, NY: McGraw. 2012: 1097–1118.

REVIEWS (FREE TEXT AVAILABLE ON PUBMED)

Aranda-Narváez JM, González-Sánchez AJ, Montiel-Casado MC, Titos-García A, Santoyo- Santoyo J. Acute necrotizing pancreatitis: Surgical indications and technical procedures. *World J Clin Cases.* 2014;2(12):840–5.

Banks PA, Bollen TL, Dervenis C, Gooszen HG, Johnson CD, Sarr MG, Tsiotos GG, Vege SS, Acute Pancreatitis Classification Working Group. Classification of acute pancreatitis—2012: Revision of the Atlanta classification and definitions by international consensus. *Gut.* 2013;62(1):102–11.

Besselink MG, van Santvoort HC, Nieuwenhuijs VB, Dutch Acute Pancreatitis Study Group. Minimally invasive 'step-up approach' versus maximal necrosectomy in patients with acute necrotising pancreatitis (PANTER trial): Design and rationale of a randomized controlled multicenter trial [ISRCTN13975868]. *BMC Surg.* 2006;6:6.

Bradley EL. A clinically based classification system for acute pancreatitis. Summary of the International Symposium on Acute Pancreatitis, Atlanta, GA, September 11–13, 1992. *Arch Surg.* 1993;128(5):586–90.

Dellinger EP, Forsmark CE, Layer P, Lévy P, Maraví-Poma E, Petrov MS, Shimosegawa T, et al. Determinant-based classification of acute pancreatitis severity: An international multidisciplinary consultation. *Ann Surg.* 2012;256(6):875–80.

Greenberg JA, Hsu J, Bawazeer M, Marshall J, Friedrich JO, Nathens A, Coburn N, May GR, Pearsall E, McLeod RS. Clinical practice guideline: Management of acute pancreatitis. *Can J Surg.* 2016;59(2):128–40.

Ince AT, Baysal B. Pathophysiology, classification and available guidelines of acute pancreatitis. *Turk J Gastroenterol.* 2014;25(4):351–7.

Janisch N, Gardner T. Recent Advances in Managing Acute Pancreatitis. *F1000Res.* 2015;4:F1000 Faculty Rev–1474.

Kokosis G, Perez A, Pappas TN. Surgical management of necrotizing pancreatitis: An overview. *World J Gastroenterol.* 2014;20(43):16106–12.

Sarr MG. 2012 revision of the Atlanta classification of acute pancreatitis. *Pol Arch Med Wewn.* 2013;123(3):118–24.

Sarr MG, Banks PA, Bollen TL, Dervenis C, Gooszen HG, Johnson CD, Tsiotos GG, Vege SS. The new revised classification of acute pancreatitis 2012. *Surg Clin North Am.* 2013;93(3):549–62.

Wroński M, Cebulski W, Słodkowski M, Krasnodębski IW. Minimally invasive treatment of infected pancreatic necrosis. *Prz Gastroenterol.* 2014;9(6):317–24.

Zerem E. Treatment of severe acute pancreatitis and its complications. *World J Gastroenterol.* 2014;20(38):13879–92.

WEBSITES

Cleveland Clinic, Cleveland, OH. http://www.clevelandclinicmeded.com/medicalpubs/diseasemanagement/gastroenterology/acute-pancreatitis/ (accessed April 6, 2017).

National Institute of Diabetes and Digestive and Kidney Diseases (NIDDK), USA. http://digestive.niddk.nih.gov/ddiseases/pubs/pancreatitis/index.htm (accessed April 6, 2017).

National Library of Medicine (NLM), USA. http://www.nlm.nih.gov/medlineplus/ency/article/000287.htm (accessed April 6, 2017).

Index